THE SCOUT'S GU

WILDERNESS
SURVIVAL
& FIRST AID

THE SCOUT'S GUIDE TO

WILDERNESS SURVIVAL & FIRST AID

400 **Essential Skills—Signal for Help, Build a Shelter, Emergency Response, Treat Wounds, Stay Warm, Gather Resources**

J. Wayne Fears & Grant S. Lipman, MD, FACEP, FAWM

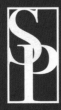

Skyhorse Publishing

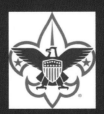

The Boy Scouts of America®

Text Copyright © 2018, 2023 by J. Wayne Fears
Illustrations Copyright © 2018, 2023 by Rod Walinchus
All images © by J. Wayne Fears, unless otherwise indicated
Logo Copyright © 2018, 2023 The Boy Scouts of America®

Skyhorse Publishing books may be purchased in bulk at special
discounts for sales promotion, corporate gifts, fund-raising, or
educational purposes. Special editions can also be created to
specifications. For details, contact the Special Sales Department,
Skyhorse Publishing, 307 West 36th Street, 11th Floor, New York,
NY 10018 or info@skyhorsepublishing.com.

Skyhorse® and Skyhorse Publishing® are registered trademarks of
Skyhorse Publishing, Inc.®, a Delaware corporation.

Visit our website at www.skyhorsepublishing.com.

10 9 8 7 6 5 4 3 2 1

Library of Congress Cataloging-in-Publication Data is available
on file.

Cover design by Kai Texel

Print ISBN: 978-1-5107-7692-0
Ebook ISBN: 978-1-5107-7805-4

Printed in China

Portions of this book were previously published as *The Scouting Guide to Wilderness First Aid*
(ISBN: 978-1-5107-3971-0) and *The Scouting Guide to Survival* (ISBN: 978-1-5107-3774-7).

CONTENTS

PART I: WILDERNESS SURVIVAL

PART II: FIRST AID

DISCLAIMER

It is the responsibility of the reader to take a wilderness first aid or equivalent training course, as the information contained in this book is not intended as a substitution for a course or practical experience. To the fullest extent of the law, neither the Author nor the Publisher assumes any liability for any injury, disability, death, and/or damage to persons or property resulting from any use or operation of any methods, products, instructions, or ideas contained in the material herein.

PART I

WILDERNESS SURVIVAL

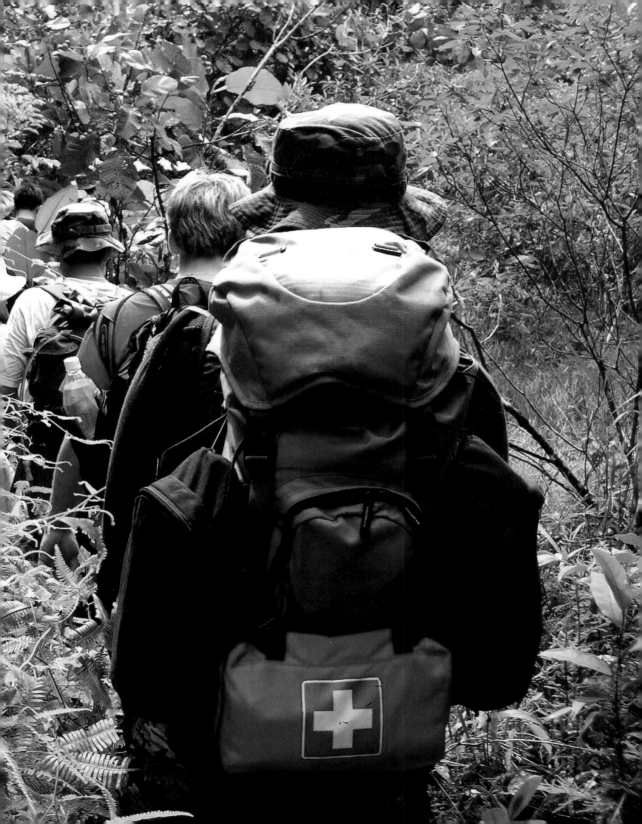

INTRODUCTION

Each year hundreds of American outdoor enthusiasts find themselves in an unexpected outdoor emergency. They get lost, injured, or stranded and suddenly find themselves cut off from the rest of the world. They suddenly have to depend upon their survival skills to survive. For most people, thanks to modern communications such as cell phones, satellite messengers, and personal locator beacons (PLB), it is merely a sobering two- or three-hour adventure. In fact, with today's high-tech methods of search and rescue, the majority of missing people are found within twenty-four hours, some a sobering seventy-two hours, after they have been reported missing. However, for some who did not take the proper precautions before they left home or do not have survival skills, it can end in tragedy.

Anyone who travels into the backcountry areas near home or deep into the wilderness needs a good working knowledge of basic survival skills. Also, those who travel through, or fly over, unpopulated areas need survival skills. The same can be said for those who venture out onto large bodies of water. Chances are good they will never become stranded in these situations, but if it happens to you, then it is a 100 percent chance.

One of the first questions I hear when conducting survival seminars is this: "Why should anyone learn survival skills?" Then they challenge: "This is the twenty-first century. Wilderness survival is no longer needed."

Few people go into a state park, national forest, or even the woods behind their home expecting to need survival skills. That "it-will-never-happen-to-me" attitude gets untold numbers of people into serious trouble each year. All too often they are found dead near snowbound automobiles, in desert sands, on mountain slopes, near downed aircraft, and in the woods near their homes. They succumb to hypothermia, are struck by lightning, or drown in flash floods. Many panic and start running, often over cliffs. Sometimes they simply lie down and die because of overwhelming fear and the lack of the will to live.

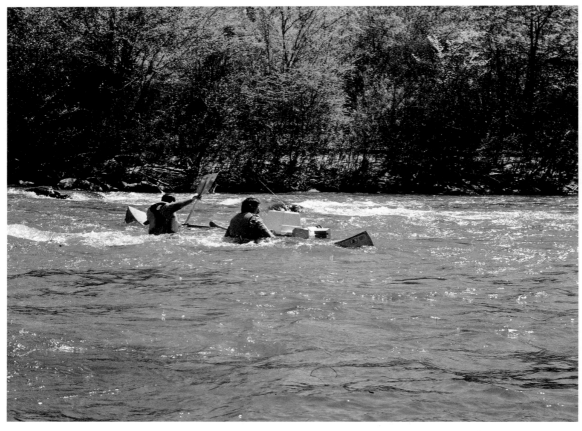

A canoe overturn in swift water can leave the occupants in a survival situation quickly.

A vast majority of people in our technological society think they will never find themselves suddenly cut off from the rest of the world. But the news media often carry stories about people who suffer and die because they don't have even the basic survival skills to keep themselves alive in an emergency. The truth is, a survival crisis can confront anyone suddenly, without warning.

I have spent most of my life in the outdoors studying the challenges of survival. Because of the nature of my career, I've seen both sides of the coin. I have been caught in severe survival situations, and have been on many search-and-rescue missions. Much of what I have learned is in this book.

This book takes to heart the Boy Scout motto of *Be Prepared!* In it we approach the subject of survival from a preparedness standpoint, rather than a collection of pioneering skills and neat tricks that you can't remember, or get to work, when you really need them. I advise the reader that spending time and energy building traps and snares are an unreliable way of getting food if you lack trapping savvy and an above-average knowledge of your quarry. You will not find pages

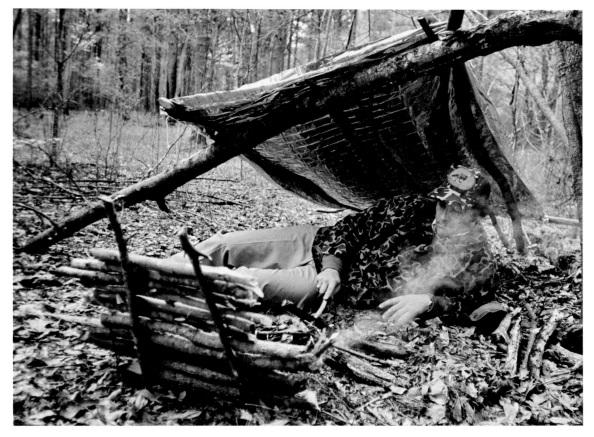

This hunter wisely decided to make a comfortable camp and await rescue rather than attempt to walk out.

of flowering wild plants that are edible because they may not grow where you find yourself in an emergency, and if they do it would probably be in the dead of winter when the plant would be impossible to identify or locate.

This book takes a realistic approach to the subject of survival. Throughout, I stress preparing for the unexpected, beginning before you leave home. My aim is to prepare you, both physically and mentally, to survive those critical first seventy-two hours. The keys are to learn that an emergency can befall you and then know what to do. I hope you will encourage other members of your troop, Explorer Post, family, and friends to learn these skills as well.

The survival training I received from both the Army and the Air Force emphasized eight basic points of survival that have helped get me through many survival situations. As a memory jog, the following acrostic, using the word SURVIVAL, helps in recalling these points, several of which appear over and over again in this book.

Size up the situation
Undue haste makes waste
Remember where you are
Vanquish fear and panic
Improvise
Value living
Act like the natives
Learn basic survival skills

SURVIVAL TRAINING PAYS

Several years ago, when I was working as a wildlife manager in Georgia, I helped lead a search for a missing hunter in the rugged mountains along the Georgia-North Carolina boundary. We were told that this hunter had little hunting experience but had received extensive survival training. In a blinding rainstorm, it took us two days to find the lost hunter. Much to our surprise, when we found him he had almost established a comfortable homestead.

When he first realized he was lost, he stopped walking and picked an opening in the dense woods to establish a survival camp. He immediately put out ground-to-air signals. Realizing bad weather was on the way, he built a shelter under some overhanging rocks that kept him dry and out of the wind. He gathered plenty of firewood and stored it in his shelter. Next, he built a fire, complete with a green log reflector, to keep his shelter warm. It was his fire that led to his being found. The hunter's survival camp was so comfortable that those of us in the search team used it for an overnight rest before packing out the next morning.

Due to his survival training, he lived comfortably through a two-day storm. He stayed positive and worked toward being found. He used the resources at hand to make a survival camp. Will you be like this hunter if your time to spend an unplanned night or two in the woods comes?

HOW TO USE THIS BOOK

1. When you first get this book, sit down and READ it. Think about what you are reading and how it can apply to you and your outings.
2. Reread the chapter on making your survival kit and make a list of the items you need to purchase to put together your own survival kit.
3. On a weekend when you want to do something that is fun and educational, take your survival kit into the woods and spend the night using the items in the kit. Upon completion of the overnight test, be sure to replace any items that may be difficult to repack into a compact package. This exercise may suggest items you will want in your survival kit that my list did not include. Remember it is YOUR survival kit, so modify it to meet your needs.
4. This book does not go into navigational skills. I feel this requires training that, like first aid, you should have before you start going into the backcountry. If you haven't had training in the proper use of your GPS and map and compass, get it ASAP. Learn to use both to travel cross country. It can keep you from ever needing this book.

5. This book does not go into first-aid skills. It is my belief that everyone who ventures into the backcountry should have successfully taken a Red Cross first aid course. Also, those who have special medical conditions should be skilled in handling them in remote emergencies.

6. Be sure to you always practice the information found in the chapter titled "Before You Go." This will keep your time in a survival situation short.

7. If you find yourself in a lost or stranded situation, stop, sit down, think, remain calm, don't panic, and plan to stay put. By getting control of yourself in these first few minutes, you have increased your survival chances by 50 percent.

8. When you first realize you are in trouble is the time to STOP!

9. As a Maine game warden once said, "Even in today's modern world, there are many trappers and guides who spend the night in the woods with little more than what is found in a basic survival kit. They spend their lives doing it. Relax. You may even enjoy your unplanned stay in the woods."

Finally, the purpose of this book is to help you prepare for that "unplanned night or nights in the woods." With the proper preparation for an outdoor activity, there should be little reason for a survival emergency. But if it should be your time to have to survive several days, this book will have you prepared to do it with style. Survival knowledge and training pays off when the chips are down. Remember, the best survival kit you have is your mind. Feed it survival knowledge, and it will be ready when that knowledge is needed.

Be Prepared!

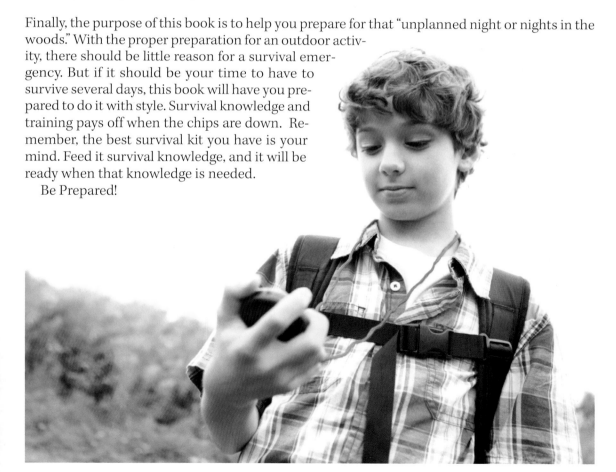

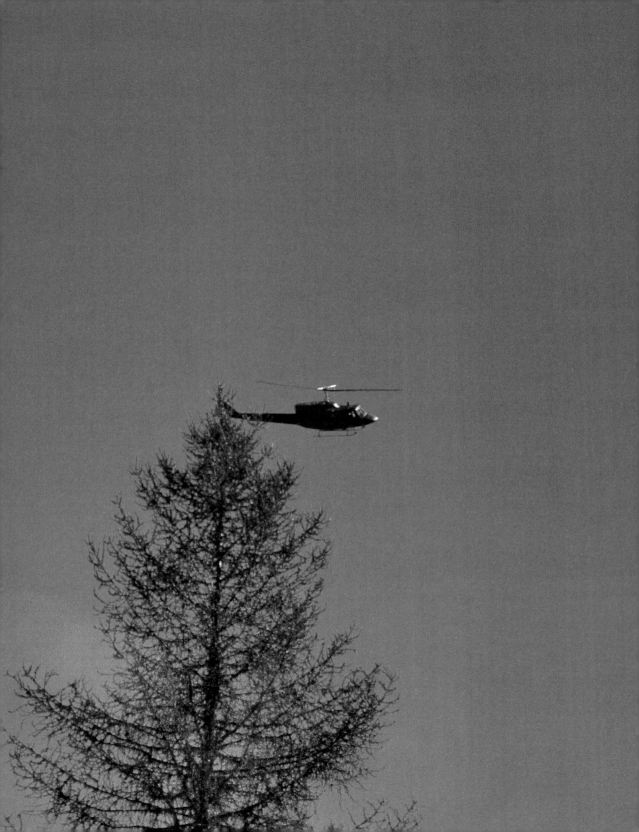

1

RESCUE IS USUALLY QUICK

With today's means of communications and transportation, few emergencies go unnoticed for long. Once the word goes out that a person is missing, even in remote areas search crews usually arrive on the scene within a few hours.

SEARCH AND RESCUE SATELLITE AIDED TRACKING

Around the world . . . around the clock . . . the National Oceanic and Atmospheric Administration (NOAA) stands watch. As an integral part of worldwide search and rescue, NOAA operates the Search and Rescue Satellite Aided Tracking (SARSAT) system to detect and locate mariners, aviators, and recreational enthusiasts with Personal Locator Beacons (PLB) in distress almost anywhere in the world, at any time, and in almost any condition.

The SARSAT system uses NOAA satellites in low-earth and geostationary orbits as well as GPS satellites in medium-earth orbit to detect and locate aviators, mariners, and land-based users in distress. The satellites relay distress signals from emergency beacons to a network of ground stations and ultimately to the US Mission Control Center (USMCC) in Suitland, Maryland. The USMCC processes the distress signal and alerts the appropriate search-and-rescue authorities to who is in distress and, more important, where they are located. Truly, SARSAT takes the "search" out of search and rescue!

Individual situations such as plane crashes, automobile breakdowns, snakebites, stranded boats, or missing persons are usually brief if the simple precautions given in this book have been taken. If you have taken the time and precaution to file a trip plan with responsible adults before your outing, then you will not go unnoticed for very long if you do not return on time or if you have a medical emergency. This will begin a series of reactions that will result in your being rescued quickly. If this one rule of common sense–to file a trip plan–were followed more often, fewer people would die and most would be rescued in hours rather than days each year.

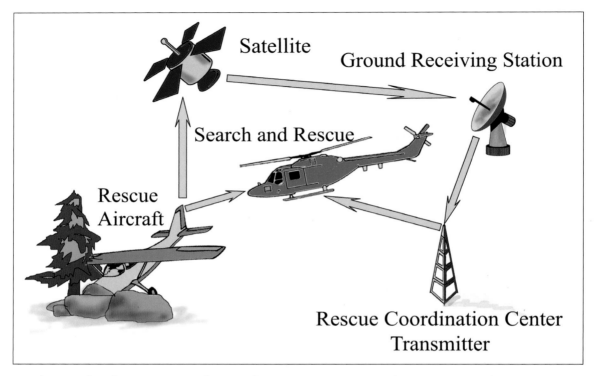

Modern technology uses satellites to locate an emergency beacon's exact location.

One of the most common and dangerous fears most lost or stranded people have is that no one will know to come looking for them. If you have followed the steps in the next chapter of this book, then you can put this fear to rest, as trained people will be looking for you soon. If you stay put once you realize you are lost or stranded, then you will be found in a short period of time. Trying to walk out, panicking, and running will work against you; it will take much longer for rescuers to find you. For every hour a lost person walks, the search area grows four times larger. You should stay put and wait to be found!

HERE IS AN EXAMPLE OF HOW IT WORKS

A search starts quickly when someone is reported missing to local authorities. In most cases this is the county sheriff, district forest ranger, or conservation officer. If it is a boat not returning from an offshore trip on large bodies of water, the Coast Guard will launch a search-and-rescue mission.

Today the National Park Service, many rural fire departments, sheriff departments, and other agencies have experienced search and rescue teams that have received formal training in search and rescue organization and techniques. They know how to respond quickly to a missing person emergency, no matter the terrain or weather. Also available for search and rescue are valuable

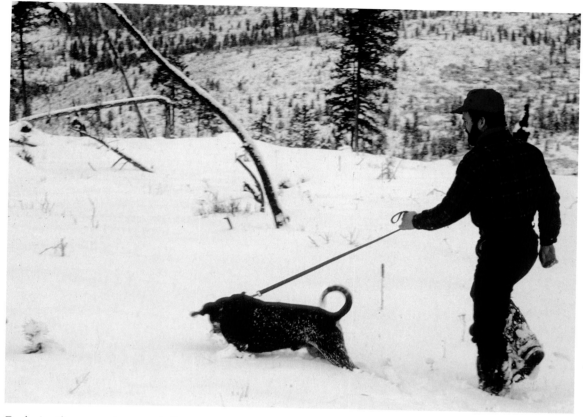

Early in the search, specially trained dogs may be used to trail a missing person.

resources such as trained search dogs, fast-water rescue teams, high-angle rescue teams, and helicopters with thermal imaging capability.

When the missing outdoor person report is turned in, the first step usually taken is that a "search boss" is designated. This is someone with experience and training in searches in the backcountry. He sets up the search organization and priorities. He will quickly protect the site where the person was last seen, set up a search headquarters, and interview those people who were last with the missing person, or who know the person well.

Protecting the "last seen" area keeps well-meaning people from destroying tracks and important signs that expert trackers will need for tracking the lost person.

The interview with the missing person's friends/family is most important, as this is where the search boss learns much about the missing person. If a trip plan has been left with someone, it will cut down on the time it takes to get an organized search started. They will have a good idea where to search.

The interviewer will be looking for detailed information on the missing person. This would include the person's name, address, description, clothing worn, boot type (sole information is

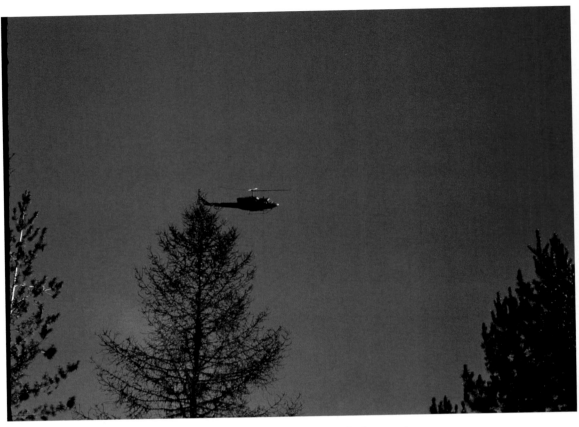

Aircraft are often used to quickly locate lost or stranded people.

important to trackers), age, equipment he has with him, medical condition (including medications), experience in the outdoors, physical condition, personality traits, and so on. All of this information is important to experienced searchers because it tells them a lot about where to look for the missing person.

Usually the first searchers on the search are trackers with dogs and a hasty team. The hasty team is made up of highly specialized people who go into the most likely areas the missing person is believed to be. This is the reason to stay put when you first realize you are lost.

At the same time, lookouts and road-check teams are posted. Lookouts are located at observation points in the search area, and road-search teams ride roads near the search area looking, and listening, for the missing person.

Aircraft, often with specialized equipment, will be brought into the search as quickly as possible. From this point on, the search boss may set up grid searches supervised by professionals, using volunteers.

Many lost people fear that searchers will only look for a few hours and give up, thinking the missing person is dead. This is not true. Most search bosses have a method of estimating how long the missing person can survive under the local conditions and then plan to search three times that long, if needed. Search efforts go far beyond reasonable expectations.

Lost and stranded people should never give up hope, for the search will go on until you are rescued. How fast the search begins depends upon how well you prepared before you went into the woods!

SAR North of the Border

Due to its vast size and range of environments, Canada relies on a diverse group of government, military, volunteer, academic, and industry partners to provide overall search and rescue (SAR) services to the public. SAR is a shared responsibility among federal, provincial/territorial, and municipal organizations, as well as air, ground, and maritime volunteer SAR organizations. There is a distinct organizational difference between the responsibility for ground SAR (GSAR) and that of aeronautical and maritime SAR.

The National Search and Rescue Program (NSP) is a Canada-wide horizontal program that integrates organizations and resources involved in the provision of search and rescue services to Canadians, including SAR response and prevention. The responsibility for the NSP resides within Public Safety and Emergency Preparedness Canada, through the National Search and Rescue Secretariat (NSS). The NSS's role is to serve as a central coordinator for the National SAR Program, working directly with federal, provincial, and territorial organizations, as well as air, ground, and marine volunteer SAR organizations involved in search and rescue activities.

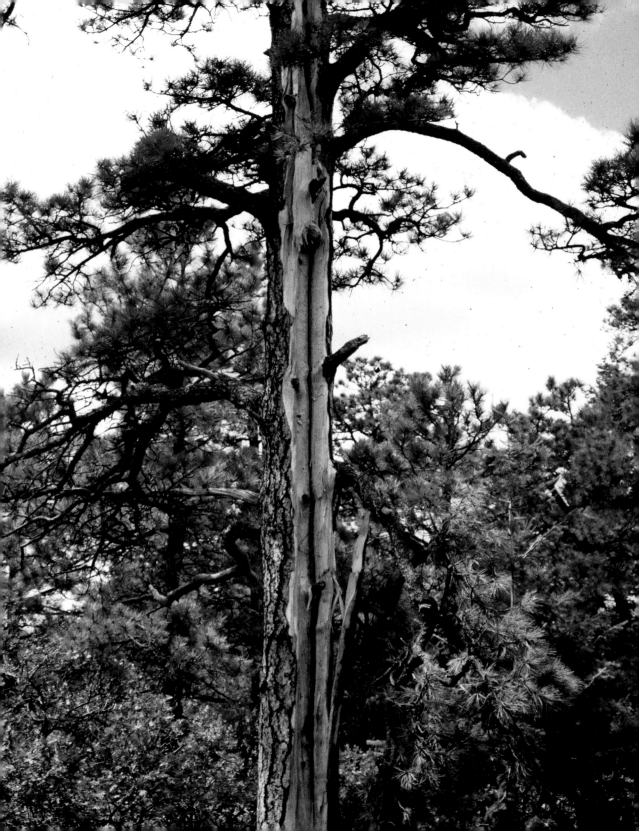

2

BEFORE YOU GO

A quick rescue actually begins before you get lost or stranded. It begins with you taking some precautions before you leave home, camp, or vehicle. Here are some commonsense precautions for an outing:

KNOW THE AREA IN WHICH YOU PLAN TO TRAVEL

When planning any trip, be sure to take the time to study USGS topographical maps of the area in detail. Pull the area up on Google Earth and see it from above. Studying up on an area in which you plan on exploring is part of the fun of the adventure. It never ceases to amaze me how many people go into the backcountry without knowing the lay of the land, the steepness, where the streams are located, where safe drinking water may be found, the directions roads run, and other essential information. If you get to know the entire area–a much larger area than the specific location you are going–beforehand, you will be able to plan an alternate route in an emergency, if needed.

Studying maps can also alert you to hidden dangers, such as streams that may be prone to flash floods in unusually heavy rainfall, terrain much steeper than you had anticipated, areas subject to avalanche, and so on. Get advice from someone who is reliable and knows the area firsthand. In parks and forests run by government agencies, this information is available from local rangers. Industrial forests, such as those owned by pulp and paper companies and timber companies, have foresters who can help prepare you for their property. The more you know about an area before going into it, the safer your trip will be.

KNOW THE AREA WEATHER EXTREMES

If an area is subject to midsummer snowstorms, hail, lightning, flash floods, or other such real extremes, you should know about them in advance. Be sure to take clothing and equipment needed for protection in the worst weather situation. You never know. You could be caught on the side of a mountain in a sudden snowstorm in July, wearing only hiking shorts and a short-sleeved shirt. Extra clothing could save your life. Always dress for the weather expected and carry clothing for weather extremes in your daypack.

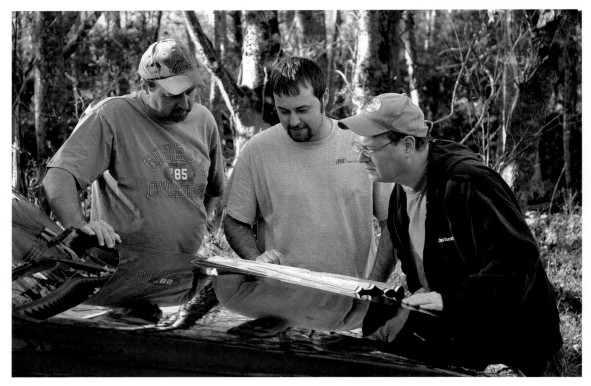

Before venturing into the backcountry, study maps and extended weather forecasts carefully and plan the event to avoid unexpected extremes.

CARRY A FRESHLY CHARGED CELL PHONE THAT HAS A LOCAL WEATHER APP

While there are areas of the country where cell phones lose a signal, these areas become fewer every year, and even when you cannot get a signal strong enough to talk to someone, texting an emergency message is still often possible. Today, the response time to lost or a stranded person has been greatly reduced due to the lost, injured, or stranded person being able to make a cell call to 911 or to a responsible person.

Also, since most areas offer weather apps, it is easy to check the weather as you travel. If you do not have a weather app, a small battery-operated NOAA weather radio can be a lifesaver if a dangerous storm is approaching just over the mountain and out of sight from you. This should never take the place of an advanced careful study of the weather forecast for the area you plan on traveling.

CONSIDER CARRYING A PERSONAL LOCATOR BEACON

For those who want extra protection or for longer trips deeper into the backcountry, consider taking a currently programmed Personal Locator Beacon (PLB). These instruments can feed reports from you, by way of satellite relay, to someone you designate, complete with an accurate location of you on a map. I use a Spot PLB, which gives a critical, life-saving line of communication when you travel beyond the boundaries of cell service. The latest generation of Spot PLBs lets family and friends know you're okay, or, if the worst should happen, sends emergency responders your need for help and GPS location–all with the push of a button. Add this weatherproof, pocket-sized PLB to your essential gear and you can stay connected wherever you roam. Just remember that the service is by subscription, so be sure the PLB you use is current on the subscription plan.

ALWAYS CARRY A SURVIVAL KIT

Equipment for any trip into the backcountry, even a short day hike, should include a survival kit. Later in this book you will find an entire chapter devoted to survival kits. Read it and make a survival kit to keep with your outdoor gear.

UNDERSTAND THE NEED FOR NAVIGATIONAL AIDS

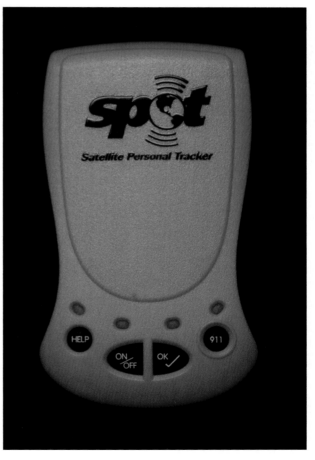

Anyone who plans to go into a backcountry area should have a GPS unit as well as a compass and map of the locale and the skills to use them. Many canoeists and kayakers floating streams and lakes think they don't need navigational aids, but an island-dotted wilderness lake or a difficult cross-country portage can change their minds in a hurry. Anyone going into the wilderness by any means—vehicle, aircraft, skis, snowshoes, horse, whatever—should have and know how to use a GPS unit, a topo map, and a compass. Start the trip by using the navigational aids. Once you realize you are lost is the wrong time to break out the compass.

A PLB, such as the Spot, can keep backcountry travelers in touch with responsible people on a regular basis thanks to the use of satellites.

TAKE OTHER NECESSARY ITEMS

When traveling in, over, or through wilderness country, take other items necessary for your own special needs. If you take medication and are going on a one-day trip, take enough for several days. In a wilderness area, I once had to bring out a diabetic camper who had forgotten his insulin and gone into shock. If you wear glasses or contact lenses, always carry a spare pair and keep them with you. Spare hearing-aid batteries are often overlooked, and if you can't hear searchers it will take much longer to be found

FILE A TRIP PLAN

This is one of the most important survival rules: Before any trip into the backcountry, or anywhere else for that matter, you should file a trip plan with at least two responsible people who will know what to do if you do not return when expected.

The trip plan should include the following information:

1. Your name, address, and cell phone number.
2. Name and phone number of someone in the area of your destination who could be called if you do not return as planned. For instance, if you are hiking in a state park far from where you live, list the state park manager's name and phone number. Having that available can save lots of time getting help on the way to you.
3. Destination name of the location you will be traveling to, or along. Give an exact location, on a topo map if possible. It is difficult to begin a search for someone if their trip plan lists the destination as the Cole National Forest, when Cole National Forest contains forty-five square miles of forestlands. Be specific and mark on the topo map the route you plan to take. If you are on a kayak trip and putting into a river at one point and taking out miles downstream, be sure to indicate these points on the map. If you plan to return to the starting point, also indicate that.
4. Purpose of the trip. Always let someone know the purpose of your trip. Is it for photographing wildflowers, climbing the rock face of a mountain, canoeing, or backpacking? If you do not return, this will give rescue teams valuable information for planning their search, as well as some idea of what could have happened.
5. Mode of transportation. If you plan to drive to a trailhead in your vehicle and then hike from that point into the backcountry, include that in your trip plan. Be sure to indicate where you will leave your vehicle. It is a good idea to record your vehicle license number in your trip plan. That way, if you don't return on time, searchers will know when they have found the right vehicle. This gives them the starting point for their search.
6. Departure date and time.
7. Planned return date and time. Try to be as accurate as possible in estimating your return, and if there is any change in the return date, notify the person who has the trip plan. If notification is impossible, do everything possible to stay with the trip plan. This could prevent an unnecessary full-scale search.
8. Names and addresses of everyone going on the trip. Include the ages of the people on the trip. Many times this information is helpful to search and rescue officials.

If you are departing from a vehicle, be sure to park the vehicle in an area where it can be found easily. Leave a slip of paper in a clear plastic bag with your name, emergency phone number, date/time of departure, description of destination, and expected return date/time. Place this bag under the windshield wiper of the vehicle. This will probably be the starting point of the search when the person you left your trip plan with notifies the authorities that you are missing. Also, this serves as a backup in case something happens to that person you left responsible to monitor your trip plan. This is an extra safety precaution

Taking these precautions is about as important as packing a survival kit. If a responsible person doesn't know you are overdue from your scheduled return, regardless of how short the trip, then no one will know to start looking for you. People have been lost for days before anyone realized there was a problem. In these cases survival ceased to be a short-term emergency and became a long-term nightmare, often with a disastrous ending.

DON'T FAIL TO TAKE THESE PRECAUTIONS!

There are many factors that could prevent your returning as planned, and filing a trip plan could be a lifesaver. Two brothers from Alabama found this out when bad weather put them two weeks behind schedule on a six-hundred-mile kayak trip in the Canadian Arctic.

The pair began their journey after filing a trip plan at Fort Reliance, Northwest Territories. They fell behind schedule when strong winds made the river too rough for paddling and limited their progress to only a few miles a day. To add to their troubles, the kayak was damaged in rapids and they had trouble repairing a hole in it. Then a blizzard struck, and they were forced to stay in their tent three days. By then, the men knew they were in trouble. But fortunately, they had filed a trip plan. When they didn't show up at their destination on time, the Royal Canadian Mounted Police began a search.

Meanwhile, the brothers started rationing their food, which for the last week of their ordeal amounted to a spoonful of lard and a spoonful of oatmeal a day.

Hoping to be spotted by a rescue plane, the men prepared a reflector mirror and kept bright items handy to use to attract attention of search planes. But when the first search plane did fly overhead, a mist obscured them from the plane's view. The plane made a second pass but then flew off as one brother waved an orange gear

Sample Trip Plan

Name:

Address:

Cell Phone:

Emergency contact name and phone number:

Destination name:

GPS coordinates of destination:

Further description of destination:

Purpose of trip:

Mode of transportation:

Departure date and time:

Return date and time:

Name/address/cell number/age of others with you:

bag. They tried to believe they'd been spotted and that help would arrive, but as the next day dragged by without rescue, they began to have doubts.

Then late that next day, after nine weeks in the Arctic, they heard a helicopter and raced from the tent, desperately waving sleeping bags. This time they were spotted and their long, cold ordeal ended.

As these two men will surely tell you, filing a detailed trip plan could save your life. But always remember to terminate the trip plan as soon as you return. I have been involved in several search and rescue operations in which the person we were looking for turned up safe and sound—down the road at a motel; at a friend's house; or, in the case of one extensive search, at a bar buying drinks for everyone to celebrate a successful whitewater kayak run. It is irresponsible to have a trip plan on file with someone and then fail to notify them when the trip is complete. Search-and-rescue operations are expensive, time-consuming, potentially dangerous to searchers, and emotionally wrenching to family members, who often fear the worst.

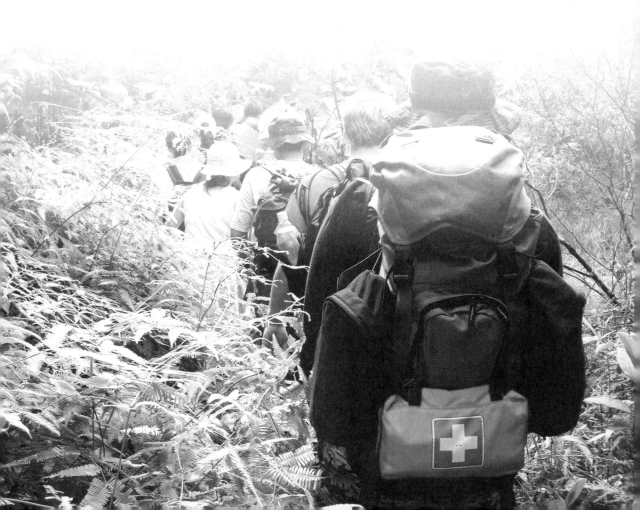

3

BE EQUIPPED FOR UNEXPECTED WEATHER

As often as not, bad weather is the cause of people in the outdoors getting lost or stranded. Having a means of keeping up with the weather is important. One of the most valuable tools any outdoorsman can have with him is a small NOAA weather-band radio. They can be purchased at many outdoor stores. The NOAA Weather Radio System broadcasts timely weather information for local areas across the US on a twenty-four-hour basis. The network is capable of reaching 90 percent of all Americans. Canada has a similar system called Weatheradio Canada.

Some weather-band radios are equipped with an alarm feature so that they will come on automatically when severe weather threatens. Most of the weather-band radios operate on a battery, making them convenient to carry into the backcountry.

Another great tool to use in keeping up to date with the local weather is a cell phone with a weather app that gives alerts if bad weather is approaching an area.

Make a cell phone with weather app or weather-band radio a must-have item of equipment for your gear, especially if the outing is a multi-day event. Use it before every outing! Before going into the woods for any period of time, take a few minutes and listen to the weather radio for forecasts of the weather during the period you will be outside. Then dress for the expected weather.

DRESS FOR THE UNEXPECTED

Whether you realize it or not, your clothing is a major part of your survival gear. It is your first line of defense against what nature throws against you. Even in areas of mild weather, the temperature can change dramatically as the time of day changes. Deserts that are hot during the day can be cold at night. Sudden rain showers with wind can change a mild day into a cold day. Climbing steep mountains can cause a person to sweat, getting his clothing wet, which can be cold in the wind.

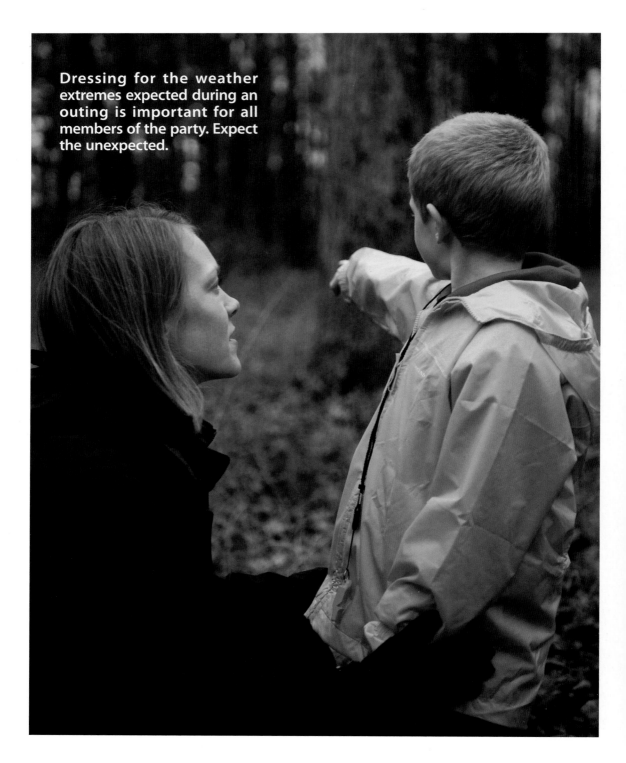

Dressing for the weather
extremes expected during an
outing is important for all
members of the party. Expect
the unexpected.

The point is, always expect the unexpected when planning an outing. Dress to be comfortable, as a specific area dictates, but always be prepared for unexpected weather changes. The best way to do this is to dress in layers: Base layer is underwear, middle layer is the layer that protects the body, and the outer layer is the layer that shields the body from wind, snow, rain, and the elements.

For warm weather the base layer—underwear and T-shirt—can be made of cotton or polyester. Today most experienced hikers choose synthetic fabric such as polyester, as this synthetic material can dry quickly and is lightweight. Cotton is comfortable but when it gets wet it is slow to dry. The middle layer might be a shirt and shorts made of cotton, polyester, or a cotton/nylon blend. Again, cotton can be slow to dry, and if a cool wind is blowing cotton can be cool. In open woodlands the shirt may have short sleeves, but in country with insects, thick brush, or lots of sun exposure, the shirt may have long sleeves to provide more protection, and you may choose to wear lightweight long pants. The head should be covered in a lightweight nylon or polyester broad-brimmed hat. For the outer layer a lightweight polyester fleece jacket may be carried in the daypack along with a lightweight breathable rain suit made from synthetic materials. Boots should be well broken in and be designed to match the weather and terrain.

If the outing is in cool or cold weather, then the layers will start with a base layer of thick polyester underwear capable of wicking moisture away from the body. The middle layer will be long pants and a long-sleeve shirt. The shirt may be made of wool, which will stay warm even when wet, and the pants may be wool blend or polyester fabric depending upon the cold anticipated. A polyester or wool sweater may be worn. Polyester fleece is warm, even when damp, but does not block the wind. The outer layer can be a wool jacket or synthetic insulated jacket. Down insulation is great until it gets wet, then it loses its insulating value. Fleece gloves with weatherproof shell will protect the hands. A fleece or wool stocking hat would be worn. Wool or wool blend socks would be worn inside well-broken-in insulated boots designed for the terrain to be encountered.

It does not take much space in a daypack to include a quality breathable rainsuit. It may come in handy on a dry day as a windbreak and, if it's brightly colored, it can be a good signal. If you get lost or stranded, you may be out a day or two longer than you expected; the weather may change, so outer layer clothing suitable for the weather encountered is good insurance.

Fabrics, insulation, and designs of outdoor clothing are changing rapidly, so it is wise to study what is available on the market today and match it to the conditions you anticipate on your outings. Proper clothing is part of the survival plan.

Dress for the expected weather temperature extremes for the period you are expecting to be out. Dress in layers so that you can remove layers and put in your daypack as the temperature warms up, or as you exert yourself. As the temperature goes lower, or you slow down exertion, you can put the layers back on.

Most important, don't go off without a hat. During cool or cold weather as much as 10 percent of your body heat loss can be from the uncovered head. This can be critical during a period of survival, especially during the night when you are trying to rest.

Wear clothing to match the climate and listen to the weather-band radio or weather app for weather changes. Don't push your luck in bad weather. If bad weather is threatening, cancel your trip—nature will be there another day. A day spent at home during dense fog, snowstorm,

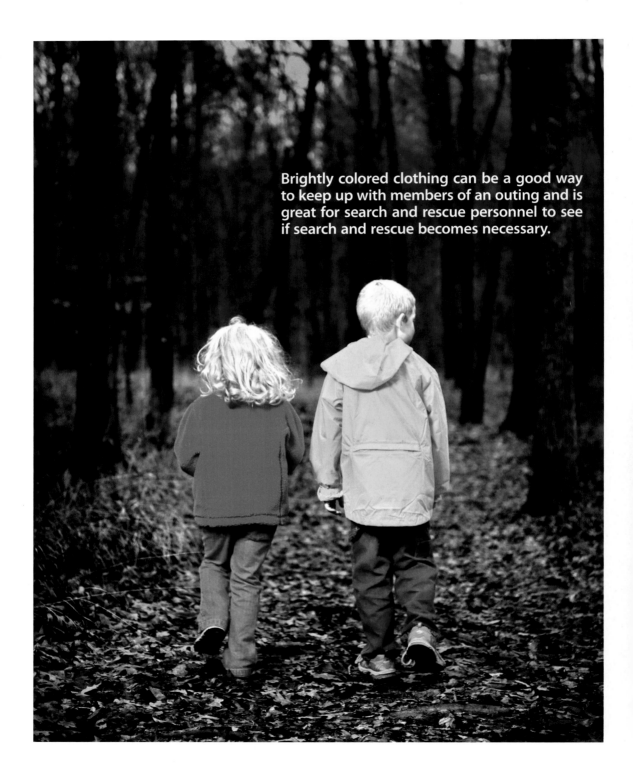

Brightly colored clothing can be a good way to keep up with members of an outing and is great for search and rescue personnel to see if search and rescue becomes necessary.

THE SCOUT'S GUIDE TO WILDERNESS SURVIVAL AND FIRST AID

thunderstorms, and so on is much better than a night in a survival camp wishing you had canceled the outing.

TAKE CARE OF YOURSELF AND YOUR EQUIPMENT

People who have been lost or stranded are frequently in sad physical and mental states when they are found. They are cut, bruised, and dirty. Their clothing is badly torn or lost altogether. Many times they are confused and very frightened.

Just because you are out in the wilderness is no reason to become careless about your body. In fact, the absence of nurses and doctors out there makes it even more important to take care of yourself and try to stay clean. A cut or sore that would be considered trivial in the city could be a life-threatening wound in certain survival situations.

Also, take care of your clothing, because it is a vital part of your survival gear. Your clothes help protect and maintain your body. Try to keep your clothing clean and dry. Clean clothing is warmer. Do not lose your clothing. Make repairs in clothing as needed.

Also, do not do what many lost people do when panic sets in and give in to the urge to run and discard items of clothing as they run. I have seen hikers and hunters who, when they became lost and started to run through the woods, discarded daypacks or hunting vests that contained plenty of items that could have been used to spend an unplanned night in the woods safely. One lost hunter I helped track had discarded his coat, hat, and hunting vest that contained matches, candy, a flashlight, and a small first-aid kit. He was found nearly naked, drowned in a beaver swamp.

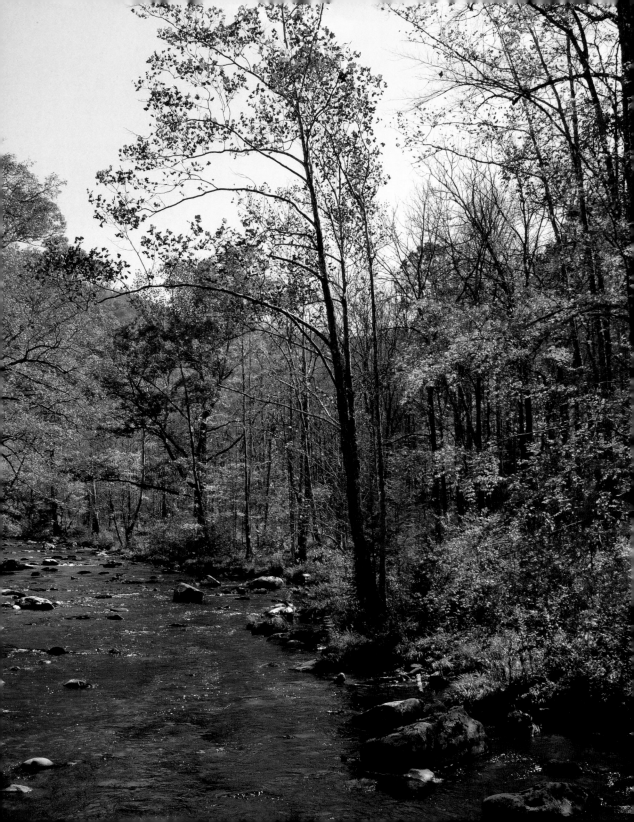

4

THIS TWO-POUND SURVIVAL KIT COULD SAVE YOUR LIFE

A survival kit offers excellent insurance for anyone who travels, regardless of whether the mode of transportation is skis, snowshoes, aircraft, boat, canoe, snowmobile, four-wheel-drive vehicle, ATV, automobile, horse or mule, or on foot.

Having a survival kit is only part of the solution, however. One must know how to use the items in the kit in order to survive. I know of an avid canoeist who carried a little survival kit with him on every trip for years. Then he lost his canoe and gear in a set of rapids on a wilderness trip in Minnesota, and he almost died because he panicked and didn't know how to use the contents of his survival kit. Learn how to use the items in your survival kit!

The survival kit is important not only for its life-saving merits, but for comfort on those outings when a night must be spent in the woods or streamside, unexpectedly. I have been forced on many occasions to

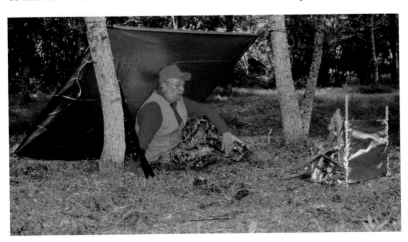

The ingredients found in a simple survival kit make a survival camp such as this possible.

spend an unexpected night or two in the woods, nights I didn't plan on, because an outfitter was late picking me up, climbing down a mountain in the dark was too dangerous, a motor conked on my boat, a glacier-melt-swollen creek blocked my return, and so on. Each time, my two-pound survival kit provided me with a comfortable camp. Without it, the waits would have been cold and dangerous.

Regardless of what type of survival kit you decide you need and whether you buy a commercial kit or put together your own, the kit must provide the basic life-saving functions for at least seventy-two hours. If you are short any of the items to meet these needs, then you don't have an adequate survival kit. The items in your kit should enable you to do the following things:

SHELTER

The first item necessary for a survival camp is shelter. You can read all you want about a lean-to, brush shelters, and wickiups, but few shelters are quicker to erect and give as much protection, especially in rain and wind, as a plastic tube tent. You simply tie a length of paracord between two trees, stretch the tube to its full eight-foot length, and crawl in out of the weather. I use the Coghlan's Tube Tent. It is compact, weighs eighteen ounces, and is a bright orange color, serving as a signal as it can be easily seen from the air. Not only have I used a tube tent in a survival situation, I have used one on several occasions for protection from a sudden rain or hail storm when I didn't have a rain suit or other protection. A fifty-foot length of paracord in your survival kit is a great aid to shelter building and many other survival camp chores.

SLEEP WARM

To stay warm in your tube tent, you will want one of the thirty-six-by-eighty-four-inch MCR Medical emergency sleeping bags. This bag, which folds up to one and a half by three inches and weighs only four ounces, will reflect and retain 90 percent of radiated body heat. You will need to be careful using one of these bags, as boots with aggressive soles can cause them to tear. But, with a little caution when getting into the bag, it will keep you warm all night. When on guided trips I carry an extra bag, as I want my guide to be rested in order to get me out safely the next day. Also, an extra bag, while weighing little and taking up little space in my survival kit, gives me a backup if I should tear the first one.

FIRE SOURCE

To build a fire you will need *fresh* strike-anywhere kitchen matches in a waterproof match box (safe). I use the full-size wooden matches because they are easy to ignite and burn longer than small matches. I keep them in a weather-tight bright orange plastic match safe. For backup, a pocket-size butane lighter works well in most situations. If using a pocket-size butane lighter, be sure that it rides in your survival kit where the gas control button is not depressed. I have seen butane lighters removed from a survival kit and the owners were shocked that all the gas had escaped.

I also keep a FireSteel magnesium rod in my kit as a third method of starting a fire. This quality-made magnesium rod can be used to start a fire quickly and easily if you have good tinder. Be cautious when shopping for magnesium rods, as there are a lot of cheap brands on the market

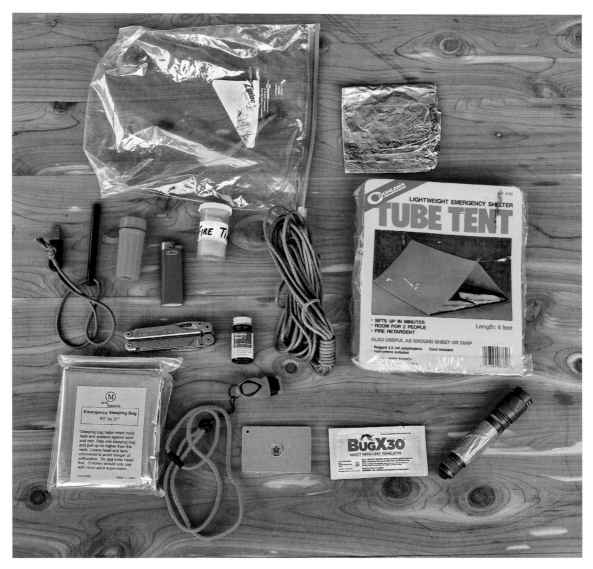

This approximate two-pound survival kit has all the ingredients necessary to sustain life for seventy-two-plus hours.

that do not work well. Practice using the magnesium bar at home before taking it into the wilderness. A survival situation is the wrong time to learn to use this method of starting a fire.

FIRE TINDER

Since starting a fire can be difficult, especially in windy or damp conditions, a package of man-made tinder is a must. While there are several brands of man-made tinder available in outdoor shops and catalogs, I make my own by rubbing petroleum jelly into 100 percent cotton balls and storing them in waterproof medicine bottles. To not carry proven tinder is to ask for trouble when a fire is a must in a driving rainstorm and warmth is critical. This is not to say that you should forget about learning the many forms of tinder that are available naturally, such as birch bark, an old bird's nest, thistle down, sedge grass, and punk, but when a fire is needed fast these natural tinders are often in scarce supply.

SIGNALING

Two methods of signaling should be carried. I suggest a signal mirror, such as a Star Flash floating mirror, and a high-quality whistle, such as a Fox 40 or WindStorm whistle. With practice, the signal mirror is easy to use and can be seen up to sixty miles or more. High-quality whistles require very little energy to use, can be heard much farther than the human voice, and last much longer. Avoid cheap whistles; they are not loud enough and some require a lot of breath to blow.

INSECT CONTROL

For protection against mosquitoes I carry small packets of BugX insect-repellent towelettes. They take up very little space in the survival kit and are worth their weight in gold during warm weather.

LIGHT

I include a small Surefire flashlight in my kit. I like the small flashlights that use LED bulbs and lithium batteries, due to their reported ten-year shelf life. A small LED high-quality flashlight can be used for signaling and is a must for doing camp chores in the dark. Some flashlights come pre-programmed to flash SOS in Morse code. Remember that the flashlight batteries in your survival kit flashlight need to be checked for freshness before you go on any outing.

SAFE WATER

While food need not be a concern for a seventy-two-hour ordeal, water will be necessary. Since safe drinking water has become scarce even in the most remote wilderness areas, it is a good idea to take along either a personal water filter such as Sawyer Mini filter or a small bottle of Potable Aqua tablets to treat drinking water. One of the most versatile items I carry in my survival kit is a twenty-four-inch by twenty-four-inch piece of heavy-duty aluminum foil folded up to about three by three inches. It can be used to make a vessel for boiling water, cooking food, making a reflector for a fire, and as a signal mirror. Pack your survival kit in a one-gallon Ziploc bag and that can be used to hold water while treating.

DUCT TAPE

Duct tape can be used for many purposes in a survival situation. I have used it for patching a hole in my canoe, taping a tear in my emergency sleeping bag, to hold a splint in place, and more. Wrap a three-foot length of duct tape to your flashlight to have on hand when it's needed. I find that wrapping it on my flashlight lets me hold my light in my teeth when I need both hands free at night.

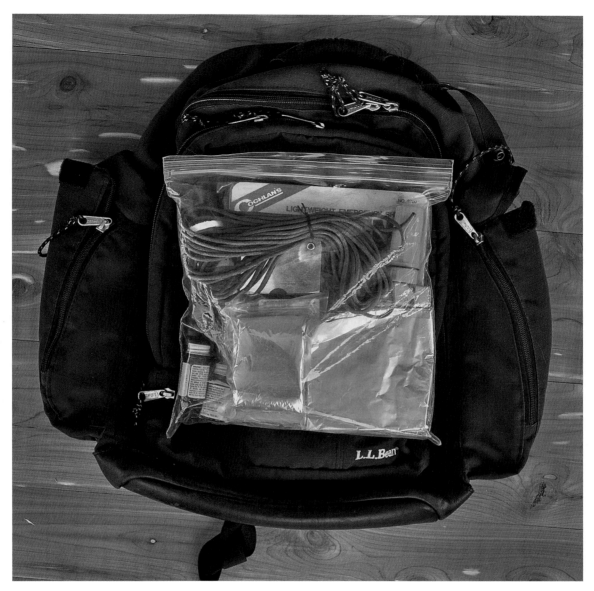

This suggested survival kit is compact, lightweight, and takes up little space in a daypack, hunting coat or fishing vest.

KNIFE

Like most survival instuctors, I consider a knife one of the most valuable survival tools to have on hand. Some people like to carry a high-quality folding knife in their survival kit. I like to have a fixed-blade knife on my belt where it is fast and easy to get to in an emergency. I also find that a good fixed-blade knife will handle larger cutting chores better than smaller folding knives will. This is a matter of preference, but a quality knife is a must in a survival situation.

It is not sufficient to purchase all these items and put them in your daypack, tacklebox, or coat pocket to be there when you need them. As with any other specialized outdoor gear, you need to give them a field test, actually use them overnight, so you are familiar with them when you need them. You may find you want to include more items.

Also, if you take medication or wear glasses, you may want to take extras in your kit. A charged cell phone, while not a part of the kit, is also good to carry.

It is a good idea to check your survival kit often to make sure your items are all there and in good shape. Some items, such as matches, must be replaced periodically.

Be sure to keep your survival kit compact and easy to pack or carry. Large survival kits have a way of being left behind. A small, compact kit is easy to carry with you.

Suggested Items for the Personal Survival Kit

- Coghlan's tube tent
- Strike-anywhere kitchen matches in an orange waterproof match safe
- FireSteel magnesium rod
- Butane lighter
- SureFire LED flashlight
- Fire tinder–petroleum jelly cotton balls in water-proof container
- StarFlash floating signal mirror
- Fox 40 or WindStorm whistle
- MRC Medical emergency sleeping bag
- Paracord—fifty feet
- Aluminum foil–36"X36"
- BugX insect-repellent towelettes
- Duct tape–three feet wrapped around flashlight or water bottle
- Potable Aqua water purification tablets or Sawyer mini-filtration device
- Re-sealable heavy-duty plastic bag–one gallon
- Quality pocketknife or belt knife

These items make up your personal survival kit. When combined with your map, compass, GPS, and cell phone, it gives you the edge you need to survive.

5
SURVIVAL PRIORITIES

Your most important survival skill is your ability to admit that you are lost or stranded. That is not an easy decision to make. Most people will not admit that until they have wandered around for long periods and gotten into a worse situation than they would have been in had they admitted their predicament at the beginning.

Once you admit that you are lost or stranded, sit down and think. If you have a cell phone, now is the time to call for help and await the help. Get control of yourself, avoid panic, and stay calm. Mentally you must accept the challenge you are facing and make the best of the adventure. If you left a trip plan with a responsible person, chances are that people will be looking for you soon. Your adventure will be short lived. Even in remote regions of North America, 99 percent of the missing people on outings are found within seventy-two hours or less. You will be too.

Let's face it, avoiding panic is difficult when dealing with yourself or, if you are not alone, with those people in your group. Most people who get lost or stranded panic to some degree, but those who fare best are those who get control of panic quickly. In extreme cases, those who panic may forget who they are or where they are. Some even hide from searchers. This erratic behavior makes it difficult for searchers to find them. Later in this chapter are the seven survival priorities to prevent panic.

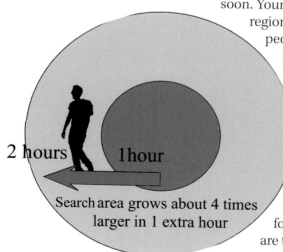

2 hours   1 hour

Search area grows about 4 times larger in 1 extra hour

As this chart shows, the longer a lost person walks the greater the search area becomes, resulting in a long-delayed rescue.

STOP

The first thing to do when you admit to yourself that you are lost or stranded is to resist the temptation to walk or run your way out of the situation. STOP! This is the acronym for:

Sit
Think
Observe
Plan

Follow this simple plan of controlling panic.

Sit: The act of sitting down will help keep you from getting into deeper trouble. This one act alone can also start the thinking process, and it helps suppress the urge to run or to make hasty, foolish decisions. You will need this time to get over the shock that it has happened to you: YOU ARE LOST.

Think: Survival is the challenge to stay alive. Your mind is the best survival kit you have. In a survival situation, you are at the mercy of your mind. In order to survive, you must keep control of your mind by thinking of past training, by maintaining a positive mental attitude, and by determination.

Think about what survival instructors call the Rules of Three:

- You may be doomed in three seconds if you let panic rule.
- You cannot live more than three minutes without oxygen.
- You cannot live more than three hours in temperature extremes without body shelter.
- You cannot live more than three days without water.
- You will begin to need food in three weeks.

These Rules of Three tell you that you need to think of the real and immediate dangers, not those conjured up by your fears. Your most immediate danger is your own mind. Don't let fear take control and cloud clear, resourceful thinking.

Observe: Observe your surroundings to discover what problems must be solved and what resources you have to solve them. You will need shelter, signals, fire, water, and a campsite that is easily spotted. First aid may be needed on yourself or someone else. Select a campsite, get out your survival kit, and set about getting ready to be found. If you are with others, make job assignments. Get everyone involved. Keep all busy. Keep everyone positive.

Plan: Now that you are settled down and ready to live the adventure, make plans to set them in motion. If you are in a group, gather the group and get organized to be found. What do you have that will aid in your survival? What natural materials are at hand? Select a survival campsite. Set out signals. Keep calm and be comfortable out of the weather while you await rescue. Having a plan makes the wait go smoothly and safely.

The STOP acronym has value, so learn it and follow it.

1. Provide First Aid

If you or a member of your group has life-threatening injuries or illness, take action at once to take care of that person. Put your first aid training to work.

2. Seek Shelter

If the weather is extreme or appears to be getting bad, shelter is a top priority. Heat can kill quickly without shade and water. If it is raining and the wind is blowing, hypothermia is a threat that must be taken seriously. Shelter out of the elements is a must.

3. Build a Fire

Fire can be a lifesaver in many ways. It can provide much-needed warmth on cold days, dry wet clothing, be a signal to searchers, boil water for safe drinking, cook food, boost one's spirits, and keep animals at bay. Having fire-making items in your survival kit and knowing how to build a fire are essential survival skills.

4. Signal for Help

Once it is realized that you are in trouble, be it a call on your cell phone or not returning when your trip plan said, a search will be started right away. Having signals out or ready to use at once becomes very important to your being found quickly. Follow the instructions given in this book to make sure your signals can be seen or heard by searchers.

5. Drink Water

Dehydration is a great danger in a survival situation. The body is about 65 percent water and it takes a lot of water, about eight glasses per day, to keep the mind sharp and the body functioning at its peak rate. That is the reason why we suggest that you have methods for making water safe to drink in your survival kit. No outing should be taken without taking plenty of water with you. We devote a chapter of this book on making water found naturally in the wild safe to drink. The body will start shutting down if it is not receiving water within about three days.

6. Don't Worry About Food

Since in all likelihood you will be rescued within seventy-two hours, food is the least likely of your survival priorities. Most of us carry around enough body fat to go many days without eating. Chances are really good that you will be out of the wilderness long before you start losing weight.

7. Have a Will to Live

There have been countless numbers of people who were lost or stranded for weeks without food, fire, or shelter. When they were found, they were in good shape. On the other hand there have been cases where people were lost just a day or so, and they perished. The difference between these people was that those who made it in good condition had a strong WILL TO LIVE. They never gave up hope of being found. They made the best of a bad situation. They didn't panic. They stayed put. They made the best of the resources at hand; and they had, or quickly developed, a positive mental attitude. In today's terms, they kept their cool. You have to value life in order to take charge of your mind and the situation you find yourself in. Give up your value of life and you will not last long.

Once you get over the first shock wave that you are lost or stranded, put a high value on your life and capitalize on your WILL TO LIVE. You will be amazed at what it will get you through.

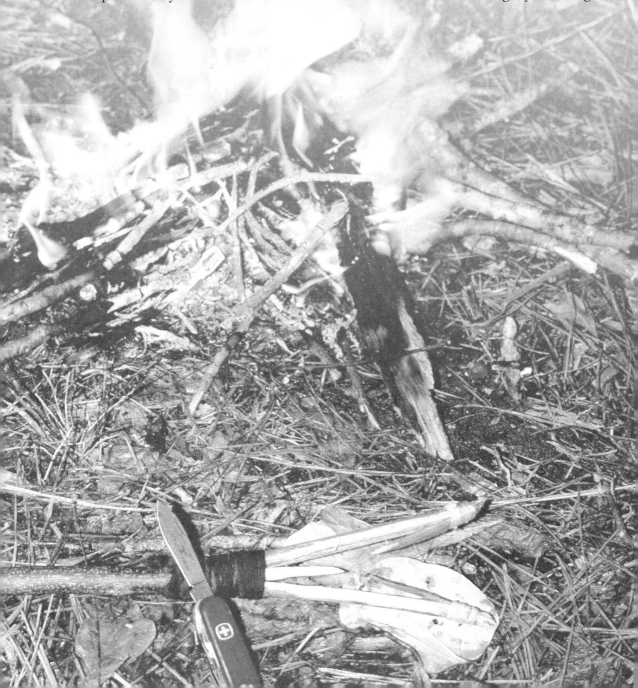

6
MANAGING FEAR

Most people think, "Survival training is something I won't need." But each year, thousands of travelers, sportsmen, campers, hikers, and others find themselves suddenly lost or stranded in North America's backcountry, often not too far from home. Here is an example I saw myself several years ago.

It had started out as a typical afternoon squirrel hunt. Three of us had taken an afternoon off to hunt in the big hardwoods found in a nearby national forest. As dusk gave way to darkness, two of us leaned on the car reliving, blow by blow, the accounts of the afternoon hunt. Suddenly it occurred to us that the third member of our party hadn't returned to the car, and darkness had now set in. Yet we didn't worry, since Mike was a trained and experienced outdoorsman. He was working on his master's degree in forest management and had just recently returned from four years of working in the Alaskan backcountry.

After thirty more minutes of waiting, I blew the car horn three times. No response. For the next ten minutes we blew the horn and shouted, stopping occasionally to listen. It was becoming very clear that Mike was in trouble. We began to wonder if he was hurt. Mike was a very safe hunter and was in excellent physical condition, so any questions along those lines seemed to be out of place. The reality that Mike was lost began to sink in. Shortly thereafter, an organized search began.

An hour after midnight, a wild-looking man broke through a thicket and ran into the light cast by the searchers' spotlights. Mike was wide-eyed and confused. His clothing from the waist down was torn to shreds and his legs and arms were bloody from the mass of scratches he had received. The .22 rifle, hunting coat, and cap he had taken into the woods with him were gone, where he did not know. We later learned that his coat contained matches, extra ammunition, a pocketknife, and three squirrels, enough survival items to live comfortably for many days.

It took Mike two weeks to fully recover from his brief but brutal ordeal. He recalled the panic that struck him at dark when he realized he was lost. He remembered running for long periods of time. He also remembered a feeling of fear toward the strange people shouting and flashing lights in the woods. The feelings of embarrassment, guilt, confusion, and exhaustion all raced through his mind at the same time. Mike, an above-average outdoorsman, had come face to face with a survival situation and had not used the skills to live.

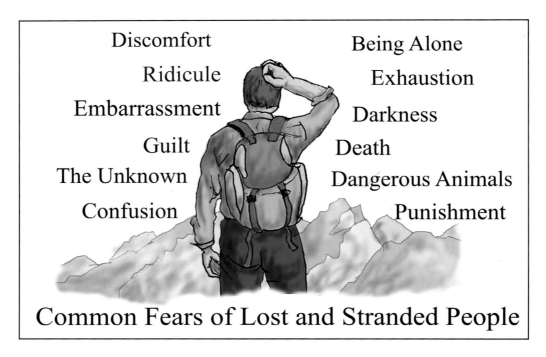

Discomfort	Being Alone
Ridicule	Exhaustion
Embarrassment	Darkness
Guilt	Death
The Unknown	Dangerous Animals
Confusion	Punishment

Common Fears of Lost and Stranded People

One of the first reactions to being lost or stranded in the backcountry is fear. It is fear that causes many people to panic soon after they realize that they are in a survival situation. It was fear that made Mike run blindly in the dark and discard his equipment.

CAUSES OF FEAR

Here is what research has shown that most people fear in a survival situation:

1. Ridicule or embarrassment: Those I have interviewed soon after rescue said this was the first fear they experienced. This is especially a major fear of experienced outdoorsmen who want to maintain their "Daniel Boone" image.
2. Punishment: It is this fear that causes many lost children and senior citizens to hide soon after they realize they are lost. Coupled with this fear is the fear of being late. Most of us live as slaves to a clock, and when we aren't where we are supposed to be, when we are supposed to be there, we face some form of punishment. This fear of punishment is present in every survival situation.
3. Being alone: Many people have never been truly alone. To them this is a strange and suddenly frightening experience. I once led a small search team for an experienced worldwide hunter. While he was only lost for a few hours, this man was in shock, as he had never been alone except in a room or other such circumstance. In his travels all over the world, he was always with a guide or group. The few hours he spent lost, alone, caused him to end his hunting career.

4. Animals: Many people have hidden fears of wild animals and sounds in the woods. In my military career, I saw some of the best trained fighters in the world who were frightened of wild animals to the point of becoming less proficient than they could have been. The fear of wild animals is mentioned by many formerly lost and stranded people, especially children. Most people forget under the stress of survival that wild animals prefer to avoid people and, with the exception of an occasional bear or mountain lion, wild animals of North America don't attack people.

5. Darkness: Darkness brings on fear to many people under survival stress. I was once stranded in a remote wilderness with a geologist who was dreadfully afraid of the dark. Each night when it got dark, he would go into a deep sleep and stay in this state of sleep until daylight. Nothing could wake him. In the dark there are sounds which sound menacing and awful and bring on fear. I have heard a beetle crawling in dry leaves sound like an animal weighing one hundred pounds crawling. The night brings out the worst in our imaginations and scares some people to the extreme.

6. The unknown: Coupled with the fear of darkness is the fear of the unknown. Questions like "What should I do? Will anyone look for me? What's that strange noise?" fill the mind of a person under survival stress. Research also shows that people tend to magnify the unknown. The less the mind has to occupy it, the more it will be plagued with the fear of the unknown.

7. Death: Death is something very few people think of or face very often. However, in a survival situation, death is suddenly on the mind. Once in an extreme survival situation in Canada, I saw a man cry and repeat over and over, "I will never see my wife and children again." With this kind of thinking, the will to live cannot enter the mind and death can come about. The fear of death can paralyze one who is not even in a life-threatening situation.

8. Discomfort: This is one of the most common fears. Survival means little rest, sleeping on the ground, drinking muddy water, insect bites, cold, heat, and many other uncomfortable things. While usually not serious, many people in our modern world cannot cope with these possible discomforts and instead panic. Many times, with a little calm thinking, most of these discomforts could be avoided.

9. Ignorance: With proper training, this is one of the fears that could be avoided. This fear is the one that causes the lost person to say, "I don't know the first thing to do. I'm in big trouble!" His first reaction is to run away from the problem. This gets him into more trouble.

Fear may vary widely in intensity, duration, and frequency of occurrence, with effects on behavior ranging from mild discomfort to complete disorganization and panic. Fear may control your behavior, and you may react to your feelings and imagination rather than to the problem that caused the fear. The situations you face in survival are, however, within reasonable bounds.

SIGNS OF FEAR

The physical symptoms of fear include:

- Quickening of pulse, trembling;
- Dilation of pupils;
- Increased muscular tension and fatigue;
- Perspiration of palms of hands, soles of feet, and armpits;
- Dryness of mouth and throat, higher pitch of voice, stammering;
- Feeling of "butterflies in stomach" and emptiness of stomach, faintness, and nausea.

Accompanying these physical symptoms, the following psychological symptoms are common:

- Irritability, increased hostility;
- Talkativeness in early stages, leading finally to speechlessness;
- Confusion, forgetfulness, and inability to concentrate;
- Feelings of unreality, flight, panic, or stupor.

SUGGESTIONS FOR CONTROLLING FEAR

Many of us have come to consider comfort as our greatest need. Comfort is not essential, and we often value it much too highly when the alternative is survival. You must value your life more than your comfort and be willing to tolerate heat, hunger, dirt, itching, pain, and almost any discomfort. If you expose yourself to a bitter cold wind because you have swollen ankles and think you can't walk to the shelter of nearby timber, you have your priorities out of order. The key to this change of attitude is the reason that identifies the pain of walking as a temporary problem compared to freezing to death.

Knowing how much you can take and understanding your demands for comfort will help you endure discomforts, particularly when the discomforts are temporary. Recognition of them as discomforts will help you concentrate on effective action.

Some Suggestions to Help You Control Your Fears

- Survival training, including knowledge and experience gained in simulated situations, has the power to reduce the unknown and contribute to the control of fear.
- Don't run away from fear; recognize it, understand it, admit it, and accept it. Learn what your reactions are likely to be.
- Learn how to think, plan, and act logically even when you are afraid. Doing these effectively is to take positive action to control fear.
- Develop confidence in yourself. Increase your capabilities by keeping physically and mentally fit. Know your equipment and how to use it. Learn as much as you can about all aspects of survival and how much stress you can stand. You will find that you can stand much more than you previously thought you could.

- Be prepared. Accept the possibility that "it can happen to me." Be properly equipped and clothed at all times. Have a plan ready that you have studied. Hope for the best, but be prepared to cope with the worst.
- Keep informed. Read books on survival, such as this one. Know when danger threatens and be prepared if it comes. Increase your knowledge and thus reduce the unknown.
- Keep busy at all times. Do all you can to prevent hunger, thirst, fatigue, idleness, and ignorance about the situation, since these increase fear.
- Know how other members of your group react to stress. Learn to work together in emergencies to live, work, plan, and help each other as a team.
- Practice your religion. If you have spiritual faith, it can be a big help.
- Cultivate good survival attitudes. Keep your mind on your main goal and keep everything else in perspective. Learn to tolerate discomfort. Don't exert yourself to satisfy minor desires which may conflict with your overall goal–to survive.

Controlling Fear in Others

Survival situations such as group outings, natural disasters, stranding, downed aircraft, and stranded vehicles sometimes involve one or more people besides you. They could be family members, fellow Scouts, close friends, or just acquaintances who joined the group for a trip or a hike. In one way, having someone else along makes an emergency situation much easier–it lessens or eliminates the fear of being completely alone. And you have someone to talk to about emergency plans and to help with survival chores.

But there are problems with group survival situations as well. If family members are involved, you may feel responsible for getting loved ones into trouble. Or with acquaintances, you may not know what they can tolerate or how well they will handle fear. While you may be able to keep your own fears in check, someone else may not. That person could easily spread a sense of panic among the others and get everyone into still deeper trouble.

The following are some steps to take when in a group survival situation:

- Cultivate mutual support. The greatest support under severe stress may come from a tightly knit group. Teamwork reduces fear while making the efforts of everyone more effective.
- Use leadership skills. The most important test of leadership, and perhaps its greatest value, lies in the stress situation. Lead by example and encourage others to stay involved.
- Practice discipline. A disciplined group has a better chance of survival than an undisciplined group.
- Use contagion to your advantage. Calm behavior and demonstration of control are contagious. Both reduce fear and inspire courage.

Fear can kill or it can save lives. It is a normal reaction to danger. By understanding and controlling fear through training, through knowledge, through reducing the unknown, and by effective group action, fear can be overcome.

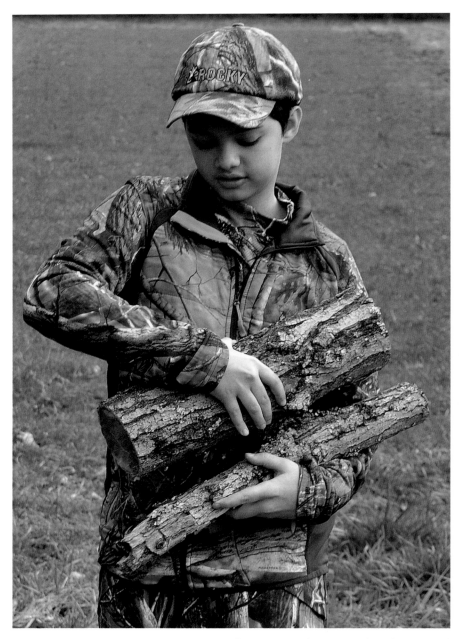

Keep everyone in a group survival situation busy. Make them and their efforts important. Idle time allows the mind to garner fears.

7

SEEK OR CONSTRUCT A SHELTER

Shelter is defined as a "place affording protection from the elements." Every survivor, faced with the problem of protecting himself from the elements, must consider using every conceivable place already existing in his immediate area or using every available material at hand to improvise a place that will afford the protection that is needed. When deciding what type of shelter to build, you must first consider what the shelter is to protect you from, such as rain, wind, insects, heat, and cold. As an example, when in hot, arid areas, protection from the sun during the day may be the prime consideration. In frigid areas, retaining body heat or keeping out high winds may be what is called for. In some seasons, swarms of insects may be the factors that dictate what type of protection the survivor must seek.

In addition to protection from natural elements and conditions, an adequate shelter also provides the survivor with psychological well-being, so necessary for sound rest. Adequate rest is extremely important if the survivor is to make sound decisions, and the need for rest becomes more critical as time passes and rescue is prolonged. Some rest contributes to mental and physical health, and adequate shelter contributes to sound rest. Because of all these factors, adequate shelters must be placed high on the priority list if survival is to be successful.

Constructing shelter for your survival camp may or may not be a rush matter. If the weather is mild with no rain, you may postpone building a shelter. However, if the weather is bad or subject to being bad, then shelter construction may become very high on your list of priorities. One plus for shelter construction, assuming you are in good shape, is that it keeps you occupied. Constructing a good shelter where you can rest comfortably out of the elements takes time and some work, but this will help keep your mind off your troubles.

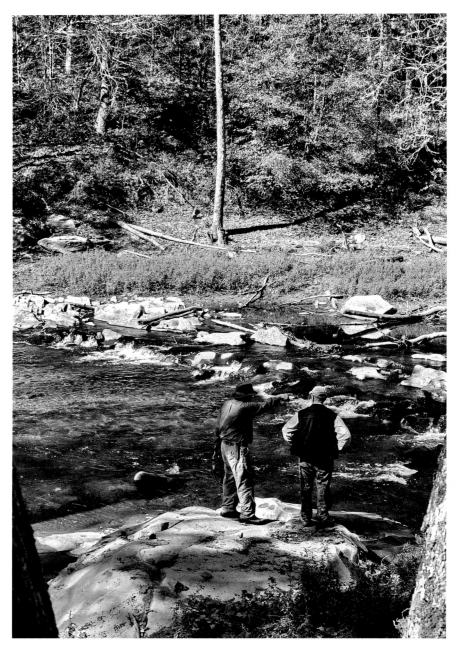

This fast-flowing creek offers water and an opening for searchers to spot the survivors; however, the survival camp should be located above the flash flood plain and far enough from the sound of the rushing waters so that aircraft or search parties can be heard.

The location of your shelter site will depend on several things. The first priority is that it be in a location where search aircraft or ground parties can easily see you. I once led a ground search party looking for two lost hikers. It took us two days longer than it should have to find the hikers due to the hidden location they had selected to set up their survival camp.

If you are stranded with a vehicle, plane, boat, snowmobile, or canoe, try to either use the craft as a camp or set up your shelter nearby due to its high visibility. The exception would be if the craft were hidden by thick brush or trees.

If you are walking or skiing, select an open area, if possible, in which to set up your survival camp. This may require that you cut some brush or small trees. Avoid constructing your shelter in a low swamp area or in a dry creek bed. Your predicament is bad enough without having to contend with a flash flood or rising ground water. Also, mosquitoes may be a problem in warm weather.

Look up before selecting a shelter site. Don't build your shelter beneath standing dead trees or dead limbs or branches that are heavy with snow, as these could fall on you. Avoid thick overhead vegetation that could prevent aircraft from seeing your shelter or your distress signals. Avoid avalanche-prone slopes. Try to construct your shelter so that you can sleep reasonably comfortably. Select a level or near-level site. Remove stones and sticks. Your sleep is vital to conserve energy for survival.

Set up a ground-to-air signal as soon as you have a survival campsite selected. If the weather is not too bad, set your signals up before you construct your shelter. To wait may cause you to miss a chance for early rescue.

If possible, find an opening and set up your shelter near a source of water such as a spring, creek, river, or lake. This saves energy in getting water. Many times such an area is visited by man more frequently than other areas.

The type of shelter you select to use in your survival camp will be based on several factors.

1. What shelter material do you have with you—tube tent, vehicle, canoe, airplane, tarp, emergency blanket, sheet of plastic, etc.?
2. What equipment do you have to aid in shelter construction—ax, saw, knife, rope, multi-tool, etc.?
3. What natural materials are available for shelter construction—rocks, trees, poles, snow, cave, etc.?
4. What is the weather like now? What kind of weather do you expect?
5. What is the season of the year?

How effective your shelter will be will depend upon these factors, plus your ability to improvise and any previous training you have had in shelter construction.

NATURAL SHELTERS

The first rule in seeking shelter is to look around you to see if a natural shelter is already in existence that might save you time in setting up your survival camp.

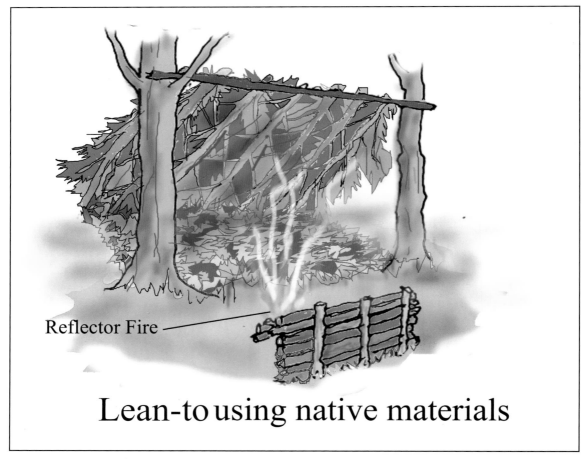

Reflector Fire

Lean-to using native materials

Lean-to made from natural materials gives some protection from the weather but few are watertight.

A rock overhang or cave can make a good shelter. In fact, during the 1700s, the longhunters who were exploring the wilderness west of the Appalachian Mountains spent entire winters in survival-type camps they made under rock overhangs. By building up rock or log walls as windbreaks, these shelters can become comfortable. The downside is that due to their locations, they are usually difficult to spot from the air or for any great distance on the ground, making rescue much more difficult. Locating ground-to-air signals nearby is a must when using these types of shelters.

In a mature forest, a huge tree that has a large hollow opening in the bottom can be used to get in out of the wind and weather. Unfortunately, not many forests that offer this type of temporary shelter exist any longer.

Many times freshly blown-down trees can be made into a survival shelter by cutting away the limbs near the ground. If large pieces of bark are around, use them to improve the roof.

If the blown-down tree has a huge root wad pulled up, and leaning over, it can be made into a shelter with little effort. However, since this shelter blends in with the surroundings, be sure to put out plenty of signals so that searchers will not overlook you.

An evergreen tree with low growing limbs that come out from the trunk and slope down to near the ground can be made into a shelter with some trimming. Again, this type of shelter blends in with the forest and really good ground-to-air signals and a fire are required for searchers to see you from the air.

If a quick search for natural shelters does not come up with an adequate shelter, then it will be up to the survivor to construct a man-made shelter from his survival kit.

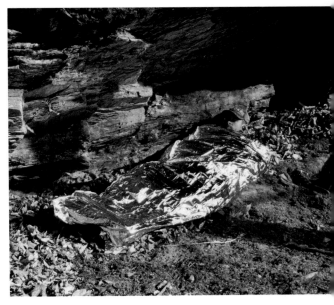

Look for good natural shelter, such as this rock overhang. However, be sure you get out ground-to-air signals in an open area so the protected area can be seen from search aircraft.

TUBE TENTS

If you are traveling in the backcountry by foot, ATV, vehicle, plane, snowmobile, canoe, boat, horseback, or skis, you would be smart to take a tube tent with you. I learned while working in northern Canada and Alaska to always have a tube tent with me at all times. I have spent many unplanned nights in the wilderness. As mentioned earlier in this guidebook, the tube tent is easy and quick to set up. You simply run a rope or cords through the plastic tube and tie it between two trees. Since they blow like a sail in high wind, it is a good idea to weigh down the front and rear openings with rocks or heavy logs until you get inside. Tube tents do a good job of keeping you dry in a rain or snow storm, they are excellent windbreaks, and due to their orange color they make a good signal.

Another feature I like about the tube tent is its use has little negative impact on the environment.

LEAN-TOS

A tarp, or emergency blanket, especially one in a metallic or bright orange color, is an extremely versatile shelter. It can be stretched over an open boat to make a cozy shelter. It can be stretched alongside an overturned canoe to form a lean-to. Stretch it from a wing of a plane to the ground or from the side of a vehicle to the ground. It makes a good lean-to, especially when trying to escape desert heat. A rain-proof lean-to is good in cold weather because, when used with a reflector fire, the shelter can be comfortable in the worst of weather.

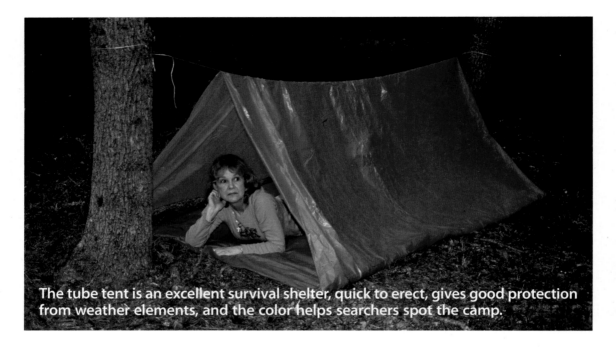
The tube tent is an excellent survival shelter, quick to erect, gives good protection from weather elements, and the color helps searchers spot the camp.

EMERGENCY BLANKETS

The Mylar emergency blanket, which is sold in many camping supply stores or by online outdoor retailers, is a good item to carry in a personal survival kit. This blanket is made from a very thin but strong space-age material which can reflect 90 percent of the heat thrown against it. It is compact, about the size of a deck of playing cards. It can be made into a lean-to, and when used with a reflector fire, is very warm. This blanket makes a warm sleeping bag when folded properly.

Any type of plastic sheeting that is large enough can be made into a lean-to. This includes cutting large plastic garbage bags so that they make a square sheet.

WICKIUPS

In the arid southwestern United States, windbreaks and shade survival shelters called wickiups are made from brush. First, build a tripod using three poles that are ten to fifteen feet long apiece. Spread the legs of

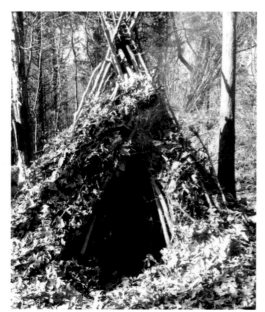

The wickiup is a good shelter to use in arid environments where shade during long hot days is important.

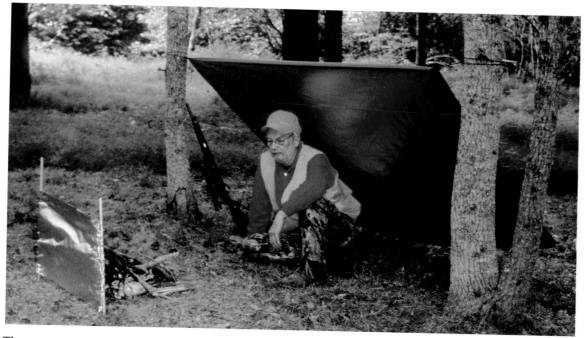

The emergency blanket can be made into a lean-to suitable for a quick survival shelter.

the tripod out six to eight feet. Next, stack long poles against the tripod until they take the shape of a tepee. Over these poles, place a thatching of sticks, grass, leaves, pine needles, evergreen boughs, and bark. These shelters are not usually rainproof but they can give good protection when a windbreak or shade is needed.

Since they blend in with the surroundings, be sure to put out plenty of signals so that searchers will not overlook you.

SNOW SHELTERS

In the winter, when there is snow on the ground, there are several survival shelters that can be constructed. However, shelters such as the well-known snow cave take a lot of energy and skill. The hole-in-the-snow shelter is one of the simpler shelters if the snow is at least four feet deep.

Hole-in-the-Snow Shelter

Find an evergreen tree having limbs extending down to snow level, then dig out all the snow around its trunk right down to the ground. Next, trim all the inside branches and use them to line the bottom and finish the top. Since this shelter is hidden, be sure to keep your ground-to-air signals out and clean of snow.

Snow Cave

A snow cave is an excellent cold-weather shelter, but it requires a lot of energy, a shovel or similar device, and some skill. Begin by finding a packed snowdrift that is about seven feet high and

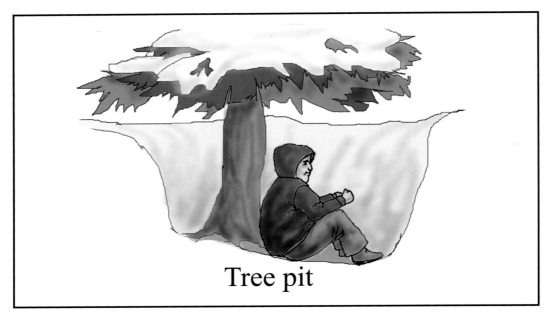

Tree pit

The hole in snow shelter is fast to make and provides a lot of protection; however, it requires effort to make sure the location can be spotted easily by searchers.

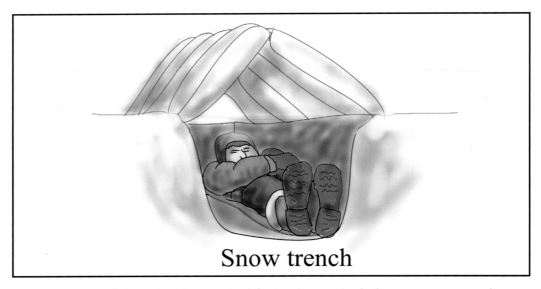

Snow trench

If getting out of the wind is a critical factor to survival, then a snow trench may be dug and blocks of packed snow used for a roof. This is usually a shelter of last resort and ground-to-air signals must be maintained or the survivor may be overlooked.

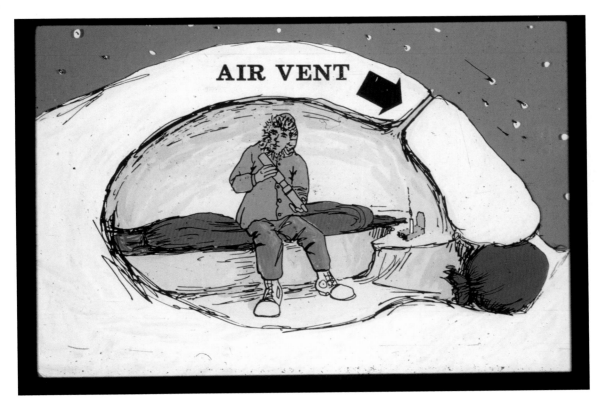

While snow caves saves lives every year, they can take a lot of energy to construct and ground-to-air signals are a must.

twelve feet or more wide. Packed snow is important so as to keep the roof of the snow cave rigid. Then start digging a low tunnel into the snow bank. After digging the tunnel two feet into the snow bank, hollow out an opening large enough for you to lie down.

Next, push a stick through the roof at a 45-degree angle to make a vent hole. In the back of the cave, build the bed platform some eighteen inches high. To conserve heat, the cave should be built just large enough to sleep, dress, and undress while lying in the sleeping bag. If desired, the sleeping shelf may be walled in to conserve heat. In addition to the ventilation hole through the roof, there should be another at the door.

Since they cannot be heated many degrees above freezing, life in snow shelters is rather rugged. It takes several weeks to acclimate yourself to the effects of living in such a cold atmosphere. You will require more food and hot drinks.

Regardless of how cold it may get outside, the temperature inside a small, well-constructed snow cave probably will not be lower than -10°F, and with a candle they can be heated to 32°F. Snow caves are difficult for searchers to find and the survivor probably will not be able to hear searchers if they are in the area.

Since snow shelters can blend in with the surroundings, good ground-to-air signals or brightly colored items laid out in an opening are a must.

There are many other crude shelters that can be made. The secret to shelter construction is simple: Use what is available to give yourself the protection necessary from the elements. Construct whatever shelter uses the least amount of energy and, if possible, keep it out where you can be seen. In most cases, the tube tent you carry in your survival kit is the best emergency shelter.

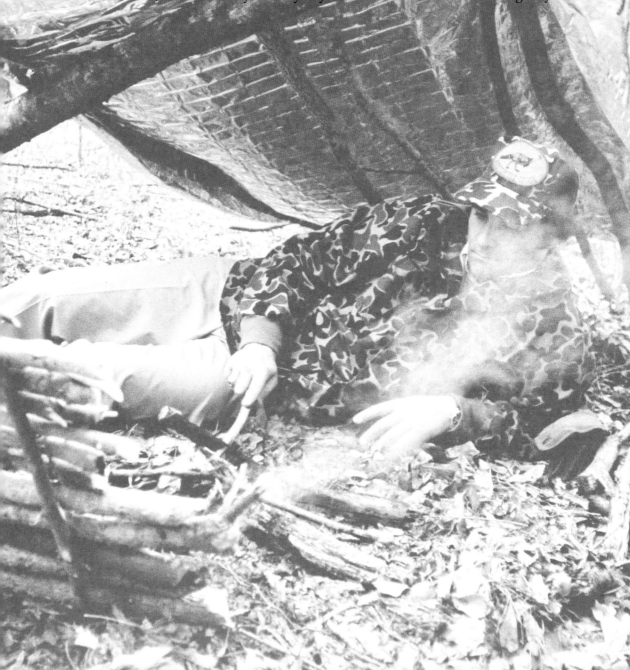

8
BUILD A SURVIVAL FIRE

You realize you are lost or, perhaps, stranded. You have stopped and calmed down. You have wisely decided to wait for rescue. Finding a nearby opening in the woods where your signals can be seen from the air, you take out your survival kit and locate your waterproof match container, and fire-starter, and build a fire. Sounds easy, doesn't it? But what if you didn't have matches? What if you didn't know how to build a fire? The unknowing might say you can always start a fire with flint and steel or with a fire drill or with a lens from your glasses. The unknowing might also say anybody can build a fire. How wrong this kind of thinking can be.

First, let's establish how valuable a fire can be to a lost or stranded person. Most people lost in the backcountry are scared, embarrassed, lonely, hungry, often cold or being attacked by flying pests, bored, and usually in poor spirits. A fire can solve many of these problems.

A survival fire serves many purposes:

- as a signal
- keeps the lost person busy
- drives away pests
- provides warmth
- purifies water
- dries clothing
- lifts spirits
- cooks food
- gives light
- may be used in crafting many useful items

Also, fire gives a sense of security and, in a way, provides company. Flame can harden a wooden spear point. Cooled down, the white ashes can be consumed to overcome constipation, the black ashes to stop diarrhea. In short, fire is one of the most valuable aids to your survival.

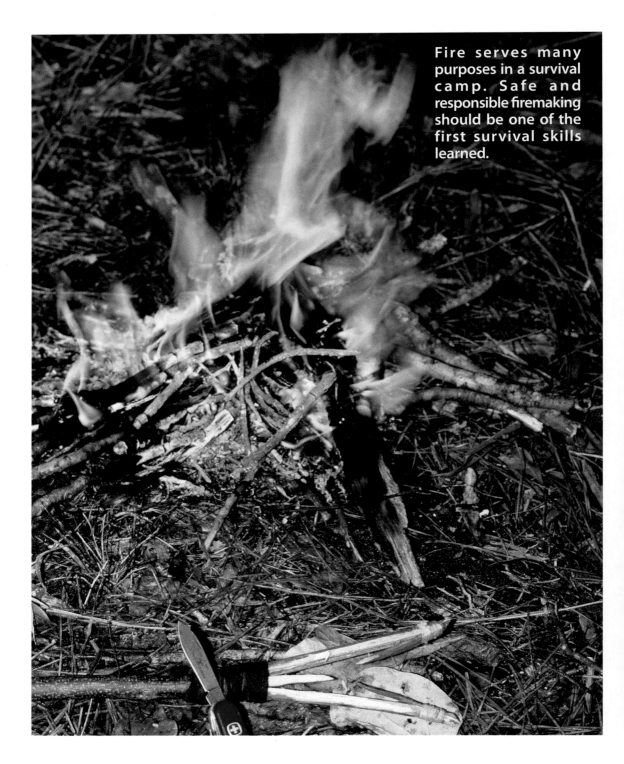

Fire serves many purposes in a survival camp. Safe and responsible firemaking should be one of the first survival skills learned.

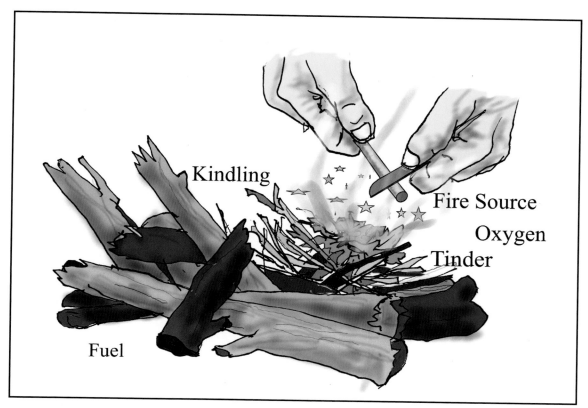

The elements of fire making.

STEPS TO BUILDING A FIRE

Understand that you don't just start a fire, you build it. There are five things you need to build a fire successfully:

1. You must have oxygen, since burning is nothing more than rapid oxidation.
2. You must have a source of very hot heat, called an igniter. Matches, a flame from a butane lighter, hot sparks from a magnesium rod: All are igniters.
3. You must have tinder to catch the flame of the match, lighter, or sparks and start the fire.
4. Next, you will need kindling–small sticks and twigs to catch the fire from the tinder and get it going hotter.
5. Finally, you will need dry, dead fuel wood and a lot more of it than you will think. Dry, dead wood can be hard to find in wet weather but it is available on lower limbs of evergreen trees, standing dead timber, or by splitting wet logs or large limbs and getting to the dry wood interior.

Igniters

Matches

Except for a few experts, there are few among us who can start a fire without matches or a lighter. Flint and steel, bow drill, and fire plow all make interesting demonstrations but seldom work in a real survival camp.

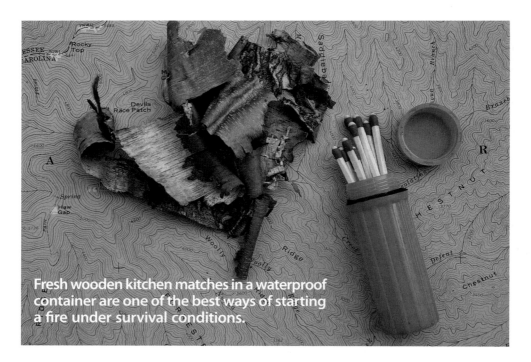

Fresh wooden kitchen matches in a waterproof container are one of the best ways of starting a fire under survival conditions.

Also, they require the use of a lot of energy. Despite what many survival books say, there are few substitutes for fresh, dry, wooden strike-anywhere kitchen matches and prepackaged tinder in a real survival situation. Make it a practice to carry a waterproof match container supplied with a fresh supply of strike-anywhere kitchen matches and tinder with you in your survival kit at all times. This combination helps makes fire-starting in cold, wet, dark conditions much quicker and easier. Make sure you replace the matches every six months or so as matches will deteriorate and become useless.

As a backup, it is smart to carry a small butane lighter to use as a source of a flame. There have been times when I have seen butane lighters have their gas release button accidentally pushed in the survival kit so that when they are needed they would only spark. Also, they can fail to give a flame at high elevations. But when they work, they work well.

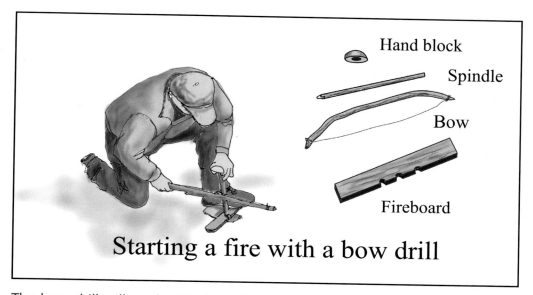

Starting a fire with a bow drill

Hand block
Spindle
Bow
Fireboard

The bow drill will, under ideal conditions, become an igniter, but contrary to what is often shown on TV, it is not an energy efficient means of making a survival fire. Add high humidity and wet wood, and it is almost impossible.

Magnesium Rods

I also carry a high-quality four-inch magnesium rod that, with a little practice and good tinder, will start a fire as well as a match. To use the rod, you use the scraper blade that is attached to the rod, or your knife, to shave off thin pieces of magnesium into a pile, about the size of a quarter, into a nest of tinder. Keep the pile of shavings fluffy and not compacted. Scrape sparks from the rod onto the pile of shavings. When the sparks hit the shavings, a very hot white flame ignites the tinder. Add kindling and then increasingly larger sticks and pieces of wood as the fire grows. Practice starting a fire with your magnesium rod before you go into the field and have to use it.

Magnifying Lenses

Anyone who has used a magnifying lens to focus the sun's rays on his own skin remembers the sudden and unbearable hotspot produced. That same magnifier will make paper smoke quite quickly, charring it. But bringing real flames from the focused sun's rays requires some

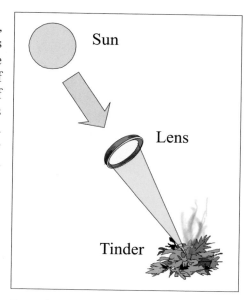

Sun

Lens

Tinder

Provided the sun is shining brightly, a fire may be started by using a lens from eyeglasses, camera, binoculars, etc.

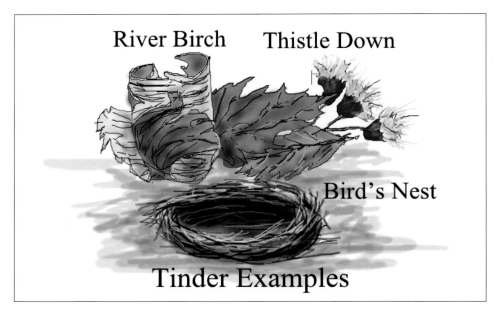

River Birch   Thistle Down

Bird's Nest

Tinder Examples

An example of three commonly found tinders.

practice with the lens you might use during a survival situation. And most important, this fire-starting method only works on sunny days.

Convex lens that you might use would include a camera lens, a plastic pocket magnifier, the front lens of a binocular or a pair of reading glasses. Before assuming that a lens will always get you a fire going on a sunny day in a survival crisis, experiment with different lenses on your chosen tinder at home first. Smoke is not enough. Practice until you can convert the sun's rays into a flame in the tinder. Once you have actually done this successfully a few times at home, then you will know what to expect in an emergency.

Batteries

Batteries found in planes, boats, automobiles, snowmobiles, ATVs, and other motors can give you enough spark, assuming they are charged, to get a fire going. Attach wires to each pole on the battery and scratch the ends together to produce sparks. Direct these sparks into the tinder.

Tinder

There are a lot of materials that can catch a spark or flame and burn easily. The trick is that you must have at least one with you or be able to identify and find natural tinder. Depending upon where you are, this can be difficult.

Here is some tinder that can be made to work. Some requires shredding, or pounding into powder:

- Shredded inner bark from cedar trees
- Shredded birch bark
- Crushed palm fiber
- Resinous sawdust
- Seed down from thistle or milkweed
- Dried pine needles, several years old
- Dried moss, such as goat's beard lichen
- 0000 steel wool
- Charred 100 percent cotton cloth
- Dry straw that is crushed
- Dry bird or rodent nest
- Crushed dead goldenrod
- Wild carrot tops
- Dryer lint
- Frayed rope
- Chaga fungus powder (inonotus obliquus)
- Dry cattail fuzz
- Cotton balls with petroleum jelly
- Crushed dried mullein leaves or colts-foot
- Spruce tips, dried
- Dry powered conifer resin
- Crushed dried grass such as broom sedge

Here is how you can make your own fire-starting tinder from 100 percent cotton balls and petroleum jelly such as Vaseline Petroleum Jelly. I have used this tinder for years and it is dependable.

1. Place several 100 percent cotton balls in a plastic pail.
2. Put a tablespoon of petroleum jelly into the pail.
3. Mix the petroleum into the cotton balls with your hands until the balls are well coated.
4. Place balls into a plastic medicine container or a close-top bag for storage and carrying into field.
5. When ready to use, pull cotton ball apart and the thin strands will catch a spark or flame easily.

Note: Handling the cotton balls is a little messy.

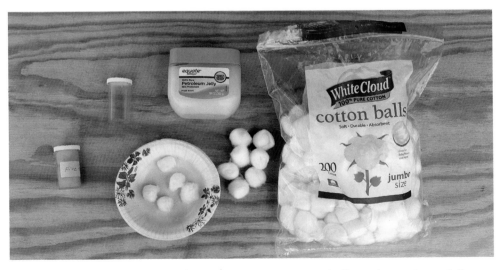

Ingredients for making tinder from 100 percent cotton balls and petroleum jelly.

Kindling

Kindling is readily combustible fuel that is added to tinder as soon as there is sufficient flame to ignite it. Add kindling to tinder to bring the burning temperature up to the point where larger and perhaps less combustible fuel can be added. When you think "kindling," think small, from the size of a match stick to the size of your thumb, and no more than twenty-four inches in length. Use a small hatchet or ax to split dry large sticks of wood into small pieces for kindling. Split kindling or fuel wood burns more readily than round wood. Here are common materials used for kindling:

- Small dry twigs or plant fibers
- Wood such as logs, large limbs, etc. split to small size
- Heavy cardboard
- Wood pieces removed from the inside of larger pieces, especially during wet conditions
- Dry wood that has been soaked in or doused with a highly flammable material such as kerosene, oil, or wax. Use with caution!
- Small dead branches, still attached to conifer trees, near the ground, called squaw wood in the far north
- Fuzz stick used to get other kindling going
- Candle; blow-out-proof birthday candle is good in the wind. Use it to get other kindling going.

Kindling should be small material that is very dry and has a high combustible point. It should be arranged over the tinder in such a fashion that it ignites when the flame from the tinder reaches it. Once on fire, the kindling burns hot enough to ignite the larger fuel wood above it. When you gather kindling, gather a generous supply, especially in wet weather, and go to great lengths to keep it dry. It usually takes a lot more kindling than you think to get a survival fire going.

Fuel

Fuel consists of those large pieces of wood or other material that keep the fire burning for long periods and may be any of the following:

- Dry standing deadwood and dry dead branches. Deadwood is easy to split and reduce to short sections by using a hatchet, ax, or pounding it on a rock.
- The inside of fallen tree trunks and large branches. These may be dry even if the outside is wet. Use the heart of the wood.
- In treeless areas, you can find other natural fuels, such as dry grass, which you can twist into bunches; peat dry enough to burn (found at the top of undercut banks); dried animal dung; animal fats; and sometimes, though rare, even natural deposits of coal.
- Even green or wet wood can be used for fuel if you have a hot enough bed of kindling burning. This hot fire forces the moisture out of this fuel and gets it hot enough to ignite. Caution: Highly flammable liquids should not be poured on any fire, even smoldering ashes, as they can explode into a ball of fire, causing serious injuries.

- Gather soft woods for flames for quick heating, hard woods for long-lasting coals such as needed for cooking or keeping warm all night.
- Gather three times more fuel wood than you think you will need.
- Keep your supply of fuel wood and kindling dry. If you don't have a tarp or other water-proof cover, use bark, large leaves, flat rocks, or anything that will shield this precious resource from rain and melting snow.
- Damp wood should be placed near the campfire to dry and store for future use.
- Remember that a campfire burns downwind, so add fuel on the lee side.
- Building a fire in the first attempt requires practice and thought. Many try to add large pieces of wood too quickly. Others try to pile on so much wood that the flame gets too little oxygen to burn. Still others do not gather up the different sizes of wood necessary to build a fire in advance, and the fire goes out while they are running around trying to find the tinder, small sticks, and fuel wood necessary.
- If you expect search planes, or are in a position so that ground searchers might see your fire or smoke, keep plenty of kindling and fuel wood on hand to get a fire going again quickly for signaling. Also, during the day, keep some green or wet leaves or conifer boughs on hand to create a signal smoke quickly.
- If you must build a fire for survival, select a location where the fire is safe and has a minimum impact on the environment.

Can you really build a fire with one match when you are cold, shaking, wet, tired, and scared? Practice, practice, practice at home! This is the time to master the art, not when it really counts.

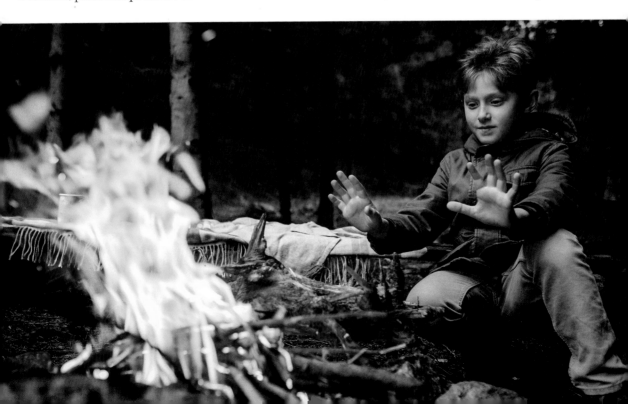

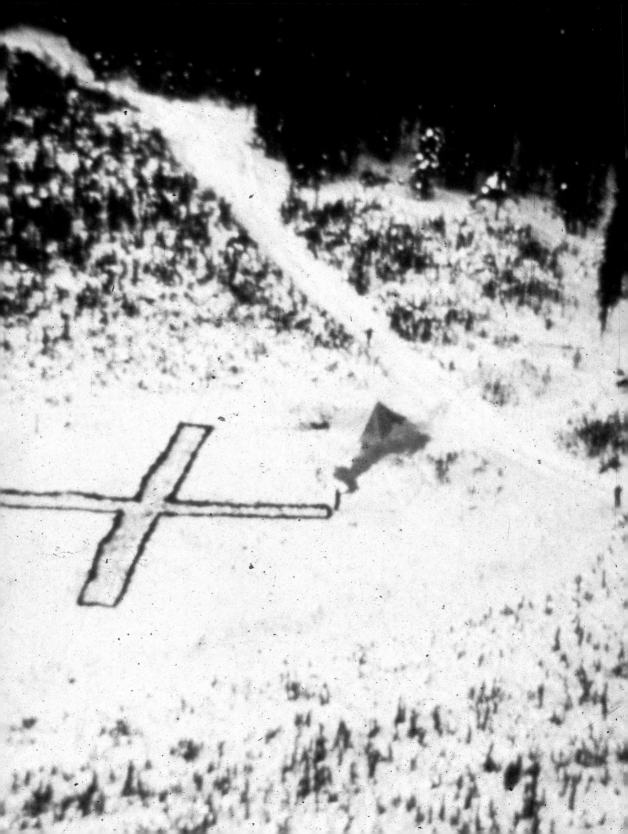

9

SIGNAL FOR HELP

Whether you are lost or stranded, the first step to being found is to leave a trip plan with a responsible person. Next, you need to be seen or heard. Assuming you have let someone know where you are going and when you expect to return, someone will soon be looking for you in the area in which you are located. Your first concern should be to get prepared to be seen, or heard, by the rescue party.

Try to avoid making your survival camp near a waterfall or roaring creek. You need to be where you can hear searchers, and a survival camp in these types of locations drowns out sounds made by searchers and sometimes your signals to them.

Signaling is a survival skill that no one should take lightly, especially since we now have excellent search aircraft that can be in the air over the search area soon after a person is reported missing. Also, hasty teams of experienced searchers can be on the ground looking for a missing person within a few hours after he or she is reported missing.

Here are some of the best signaling methods, second only to a working cell phone.

SIGNAL MIRROR

Most survival experts consider the signal mirror to be one of the best signal devices available, especially when aircraft are used in a search. They are small and easy to carry in a survival kit, coat, or daypack. It amazes people how far a reflection from these little mirrors can be seen.

US Air Force rescue planes have spotted a signal mirror from as far away as one hundred miles. Distances of thirty to forty miles are common. Several times lost people have used a signal mirror to attract the attention of rangers in a forest fire tower, or searchers miles away on a mountainside or in a flat desert.

A Texas pilot was flying home from Alaska when his helicopter crashed in a thick spruce forest in British Columbia. He survived for fourteen days at the crash site. He was found because he used a piece of shiny metal as a signal mirror to get the attention of a search-and-rescue plane as it flew over. Many downed combat pilots and military special ops units in Southeast Asia, during the 1960s and 1970s, owe their lives to signal mirrors.

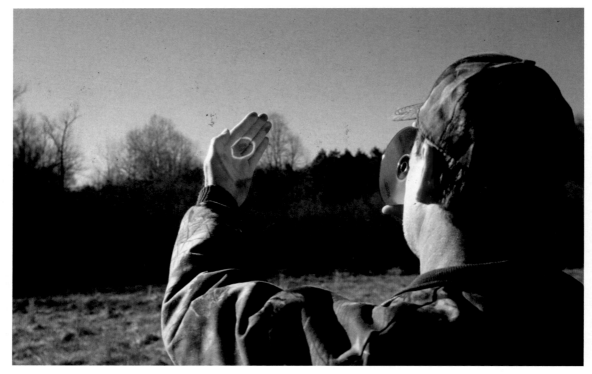

A CD makes an excellent signal mirror, complete with aiming hole in center.

Signal mirrors may be purchased at outdoor supply stores and websites. Most signal mirrors are made from glass or tough plastic and have instructions on the back. While the instructions are easy follow, no one should wait until they get in a survival situation before learning how to use the mirror properly. Practice until you understand the correct way to use the mirror.

Most signal mirrors have a hole in the center for aiming. They are used to reflect the sun, moon, or aircraft searchlight to signal an overhead aircraft, boat, or other target such as a search party that is within view but a long distance away.

Here is how to use the signal mirror:

1. Hold the mirror in front of your eye so you can see through the hole.
2. Make sure the shiny side is toward the sun, moon, or searchlight.
3. Take your other hand and hold it out at arm's length.
4. Reflect light from the sun, moon, or searchlight onto the extended hand.
5. While watching through the aiming hole, turn the mirror in order to swing the reflected spot toward the target.
6. Keep your signal mirror with you and be prepared to use it fast.

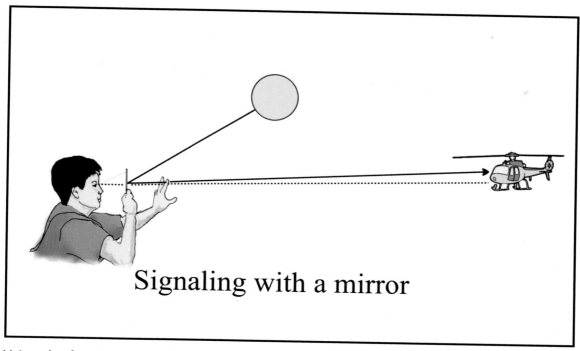

Signaling with a mirror

Using the free hand as a sight use it to guide the mirror reflection to the aircraft.

Signal mirrors may be improvised from almost any shiny object, aluminum foil, ladies' compact mirror, car mirror, top of an aluminum can with a hole in the center, or even a CD disk. In fact, a CD makes an excellent signal mirror, due to its highly reflective surface and to the hole in the center being used for an aiming device.

Signal mirrors work best on bright sunny days, but they also work on hazy and cloudy days, on bright moonlit nights, and when searchlights are used by boats or aircraft.

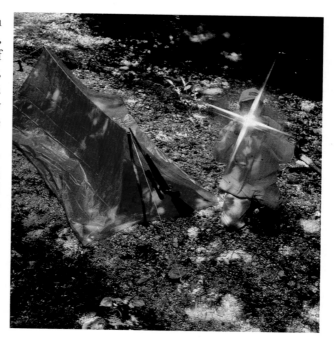

The combination of flash from the signal mirror, the bright color of the tube tent, and the bright color from the coat makes this lost hunter easy to spot from the air.

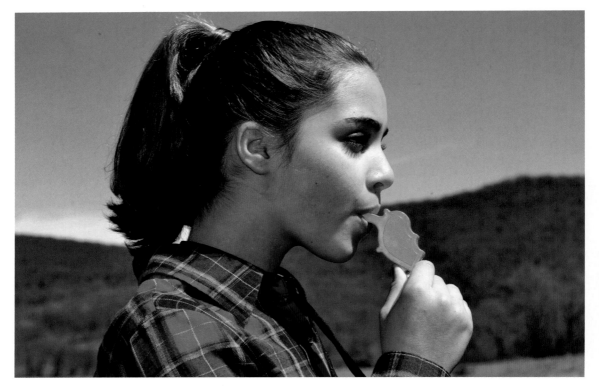

A sound from a quality whistle will carry much further than the human voice and last much longer.

WHISTLES

Loud, high-quality whistles used by military, police, and sports coaches make excellent signal devices. They are easy to carry, require little energy to use, and, at up to 130 decibels, they can be heard much farther than the human voice and last long after a shouting person becomes hoarse. Whistles make good signals when a ground party is conducting the search. They are easily heard and, if tracking dogs are being used, they can hear whistles from great distances. Be sure to get a whistle in a bright orange or yellow color, so it can be found quickly and easily when needed.

In a survival situation, take the whistle from the survival kit and wear it around your neck on a cord so that it is ready for immediate use if a search team is detected.

To use a whistle effectively, stay calm and do not blow on it until you think that someone is within hearing distance. To blow a whistle continuously for hours when no one is around only wastes vital energy and brings on frustration. When you think enough time has gone by and people are likely looking for you, try giving a few blows on your whistle every thirty minutes just in case someone is out there, and then whistle them in. When you hear searchers, stay put and let them come to you.

FIRES

One of the best-known signals, both day and night, is a fire. At night, a bright campfire in an opening can be seen for miles from the air and a fair distance on the ground, especially in mountains. During the day, the same fire can be made to smoke when wet leaves or green vegetation is piled on it. Smoke during the day is an excellent signal.

Remember to be extremely careful when making and using a signal fire. When in a survival situation, most people are upset, excited, and mistakes happen easily. You are in enough trouble already without getting caught in a forest fire that you set.

Carry kitchen matches in a waterproof container and fire-starting tinder with you. Know how to start a fire even in wet conditions. Building a fire in a survival situation is more difficult than most people think. Master the skill of fire-making before you actually need it.

For a fire to be effective, it must be prepared before the time that a rescue aircraft or search team enters the area. Then you only need to light it quickly and the fire does the rest. You should supplement the fire with other forms of signaling.

FLASHLIGHTS

One of the new generations of ultra-bright LED flashlights makes an excellent signal at night. If the flashlight has an on-off switch that allows you to signal SOS in Morse code, so much the better. Three short flashes, three long flashes, and three short flashes are the SOS signal that is known to all rescue personnel. Even a small light out in the open can be seen a long way by aircraft at night.

BRIGHT CLOTHING AND EQUIPMENT

The bright-orange clothing that many hunters wear works well as a signal, especially if aircraft are used in a search. Even a white T-shirt or yellow rainsuit can be used as a signal panel. Brightly colored equipment such as a red tube tent or orange pack can also be used to signal searchers.

GROUND-TO-AIR SIGNALS

Search pilots are all familiar with ground-to-air signals. These are large symbols the lost or stranded person forms out in the open, where they can be seen by search aircraft. They must contrast with the ground to be seen. Dark limbs on snow or light-colored rocks on dark soil are examples of what has worked.

The signal symbol must be large to be seen from the air. For example, the "X," the universal signal for help, ideally should have legs that are three feet wide and eighteen feet long.

GUNSHOTS

Gunshots can be good signals and they carry a long distance, although they must be used at the right time to be effective. If you are in trouble during hunting season, your random shots may be mistaken as shots from hunters. Save your ammunition and wait until well after dark. Then fire three shots into the air. Listen for three shots in return. If you make contact, from that point on fire only one shot when you hear your searchers shoot. Save your ammo, as it may take several shots to guide them in.

GROUND - TO - AIR SIGNALS

X	UNABLE TO TRAVEL
↑	AM TRAVELING IN THIS DIRECTION
I	NEED DOCTOR - EMERGENCY
II	NEED MEDICAL SUPPLIES
F	NEED FOOD AND WATER
⋁	NEED GUN AND AMMO
☐	NEED MAP AND COMPASS
Y	YES
N	NO
⫠⫠	DO NOT UNDERSTAND MESSAGE
LL	ALL WELL
K	WHICH DIRECTION SHOULD I GO?

Ground-to-air signals recognized by aircraft pilots.

SHADOW SIGNALS

In open snow-covered plains, it is often difficult to find materials to make ground-to-air signals or SOS. If this is the case, build your ground-to-air signal out of mounds of snow so that they cast a shadow. Due to the lack of contrast, it is the shadow the pilot or spotters will see from the search aircraft. To be effective, these shadow signals must be oriented to the sun to produce the best shadow possible. Usually an east-west line gives best results. In this case, other signal devices should be used in earnest at the same time.

Several years ago a thirteen-year-old cross-country skier who spent the night on a mountain during a sudden snowstorm was found unharmed after a ski resort employee saw a giant SOS the youngster had stamped in the snow. It was the shadows in the SOS depression that made the signal stand out.

The most important factors about signals are that you know how to use them properly, and that you have the signals ready for use on a short notice. Also, it is important that you choose an open area to do your signaling. Many of the signals discussed will not be seen from the air if you sit under a thick canopy of tall trees to await rescue. Select an open area, if possible, to wait for your rescuers and have your signals ready. Areas such as old roads, fields, sites of old forest fires, sea or lake shores, or any other types of openings will help you be seen early in the search. Remember to stay where you are, and don't give in to the urge to travel. Signaling will bring help to you.

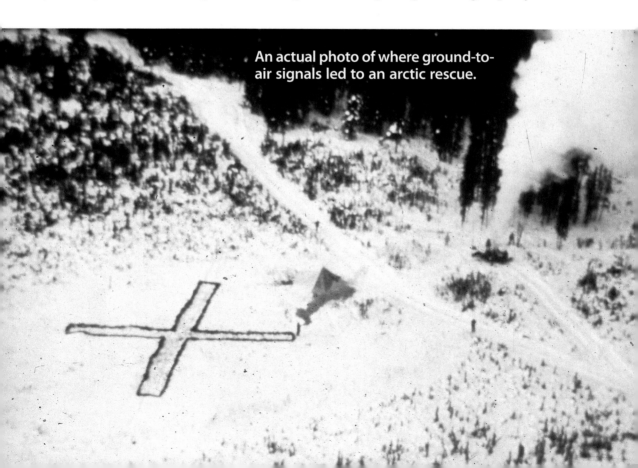

An actual photo of where ground-to-air signals led to an arctic rescue.

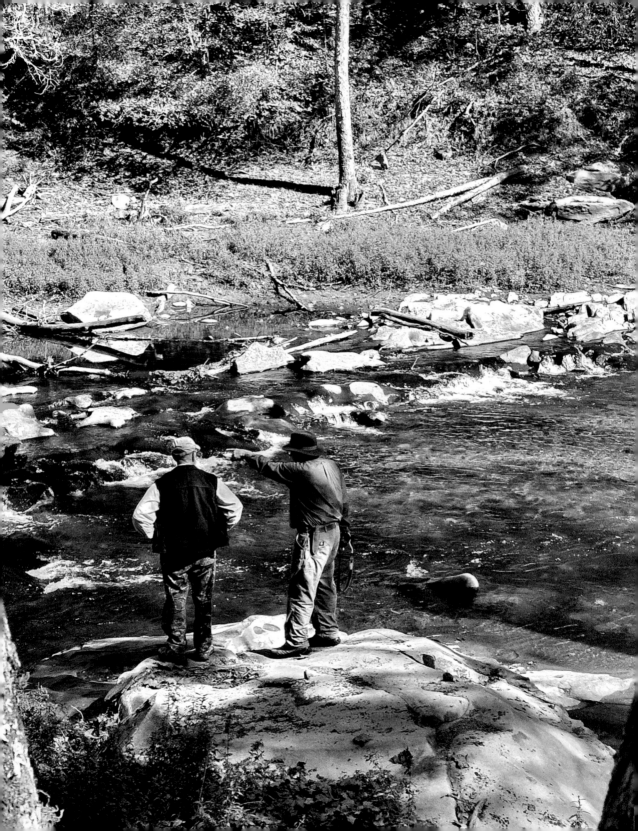

10

SAFE WATER IS ESSENTIAL

There once was a time when it would have been unnecessary to include a chapter in this book on how to make water found in the backcountry safe for drinking, but those days are gone. Today there are few areas left in the backcountry, or anywhere else, where one can trust the quality of

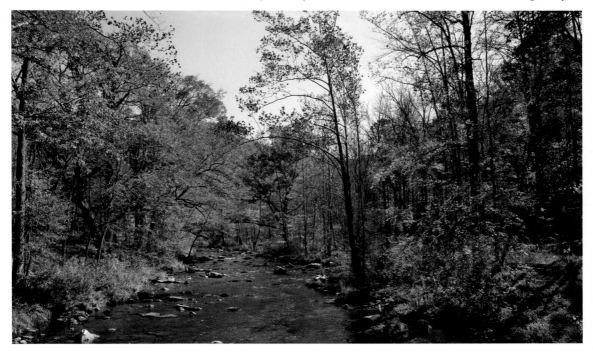

Unfortunately no creek in today's world can be considered a source of safe drinking water before the water drawn is treated or filtered.

the water and be safe in doing so. Therefore, it behooves every backcountry traveler to learn the skill of making water safe for drinking, especially those who might possibly face a survival emergency.

Survival is a stressful period in a person's life, and the need for pure drinking water is important. The body is approximately 75 percent water, and the intake and output of liquids are necessary for normal functions of the vital organs.

Daily water requirements, a minimum of two quarts, help maintain proper balance and efficiency within the system of the body. During cold weather, breathing alone releases a lot of moisture from the body. Perspiration also releases moisture. Any lower intake of water results in gradual dehydration and the loss of the body's efficiency. Losing water to the extent of 2.5 percent of body weight, or approximately one and one-half quarts of body water, will reduce efficiency 25 percent. This loss could be deadly in a survival emergency.

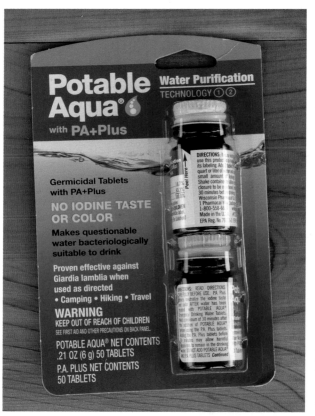

Several commercial tablets such as Potable Aqua fit easily into a survival kit and make most waters safe to drink.

There are many myths about water purifying itself in the outdoors. One popular theory is that water, swiftly running over, around, and through rocks purifies itself. Do not believe it. This is not a valid hypothesis. Another myth claims that if clear water sits in the sun for an hour, the germs are killed. Again, this is untrue. Nature produces clean water, but once it becomes unclean, rarely does nature clean it again. It is your responsibility to treat questionable water.

Never trust water from an unknown source. If you do not know the source of your water supply, do not trust it. Some of the diseases you may contract by drinking impure water include dysentery, giardiasis, cholera, and typhoid. The best way to be assured of having safe water is to carry enough with you to use for drinking. However, in an unexpected survival situation of several days, this is not always possible. It is on these types of emergencies that water treatment knowledge is a must. Here are several methods for treating questionable water:

BOILING

One of the best methods for treating water is the boiling method. Boiling water for ten minutes will produce germ-free water for drinking or cooking. Since boiling leaves water with a flat taste, you should pour it back and forth between two containers several times once it has cooled. This aerates it, giving back its natural taste. A vessel for boiling water can be formed from the aluminum foil in your survival kit.

COMMERCIAL TABLETS

Drugstores and outfitter stores usually have halazone tablets or Potable Aqua tablets for the treatment of water. A bottle of the tablets fits nicely in the individual survival kit. Both do excellent jobs. Halazone tablets have been used successfully for years. Add two tablets to a quart of water and follow with a thirty-minute wait. The newer product, Potable Aqua, requires one tablet to a quart of water, capping loosely to allow a little leakage. Wait three minutes and shake thoroughly. Wait thirty minutes before drinking. If the water is very cold or contains rotten leaves or silt, use two tablets. You can use the gallon re-sealable plastic bag in which your survival items are packed for a water container. The plastic bag in which the tube tent is packed also makes a good water container.

IODINE TREATMENT

While iodine is no longer used in some of the newer first aid kits, it is still in older kits and makes a good water treatment. Simply add five drops of iodine to one quart of clear water and ten drops to cloudy water. Let water stand for thirty minutes before drinking.

At this point I should point out that any time you are treating water in a canteen, jug, or other type of container, you should be sure to rinse the cap, spout, screw threads, and lid with some of the treated water. You do not want to miss treating any surface that may come into contact with your mouth or the water you are drinking.

WATER FILTERING DEVICES

There are a number of compact water filtration units such as Sawyer and LifeStraw that can give the backcountry traveler safe water. They have been proven to filter out Giardia and other harmful threats, and the units fit into a pack easily.

GETTING WATER IN EXTREME COLD CONDITIONS

Dehydration is almost as great a problem in cold conditions as in the desert, because all the water is frozen into snow or ice. Some streams or lakes may provide access to flowing water (but be very careful not to fall into the water). If the sun is shining, you can melt snow on a dark plastic bag or tarp, flat rock, or any surface that will absorb the sun's heat. Arrange the surface so that the melted water will drain into a hollow depression or container.

Anyone traveling under frigid conditions should carry a small portable gas-type stove and pot for melting ice or snow. Whenever possible, melt

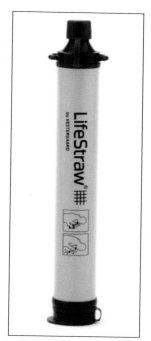

Compact water filtration systems, such as this LifeStraw, offer the backcountry traveler an option to carry in their survival kit.

ice rather than snow because ice yields more water for the volume with less heat and time. Snow is seventeen parts air and one part water. If you melt snow by heating, put in a little snow at a time and compress it, or the pot will burn. If water is available, put a little in the bottom of the pot to protect the pot and add snow gradually.

When melted, glacial ice gives roughly twice the water, per fuel unit, in half the time that snow does. In addition, snow is more likely to contain dirt, soot, and animal and human contaminants.

Don't try to eat ice or snow. A day or two of taking water in this manner will make the mucous membrane of your mouth so swollen and raw as to prevent eating or drinking until the inflammation subsides. Also, your body gives up heat to melt the snow. Dogs eat snow and get away with it; humans can't.

Once you have water, give it the boiling treatment.

COLLECTING RAIN AND DEW FOR DRINKING WATER

Dew sometimes forms on metal auto hoods and airplane wings, tube tents, or on plant leaves that can be sponged with a cloth. Some water can be obtained as dewdrops on the underside of a plastic sheet spread on the ground during the night. Use every possible means of water conservation and keep supplementing your water supply.

Watch the weather signs and be ready to collect rainwater. Rub wax from candles or butter to waterproof fabric for collecting rainwater. Spread out your waterproofed clothes to catch the rain. Remember that large leaves, holes in tree trunks, and depressions in rocks will collect water

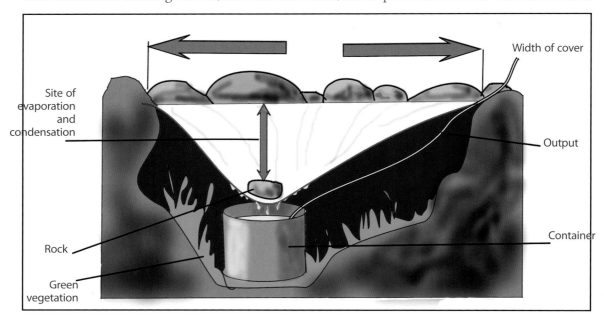

A solar still can be made in arid environments to gather small amounts of water for drinking. It does require you carry the necessary ingredients with you to make a solar still and the amount of water obtained is usually small.

for you also. Dig a hole in the ground and line it with cloth, canvas, plastic, oiled paper, or leaves–anything to stop rapid drainage into the earth.

Rainwater can be diverted from leaning trees and branches by a long cloth wick (torn from any cloth) leading into a container.

GETTING SEDIMENT OUT OF WATER
If clear water is not available, take the following steps:

1. Filter the water to be treated through a clean handkerchief or similar fabric.
2. Let the filtered water stand until any remaining sediment has settled to the bottom.
3. Pour off the clear water into the vessel; treat the water.

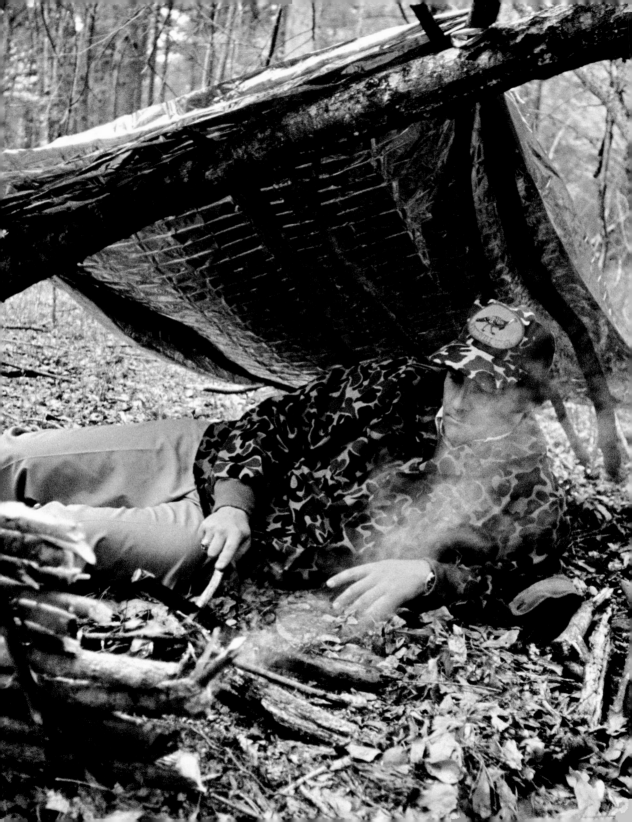

11

FOOD: NOT A NECESSITY

Every time the subject of survival is brought up, the first discussions usually revolve around edible wild foods and how to procure them. We are obsessed with eating. It has been proven many times that most of us can go without eating several weeks, if necessary, and not die. Most of us carry around an abundance of fat that could keep us alive for a long period of time. For this reason, and the fact that this book was written for the most likely survival scenario, not more than seventy-two hours in the woods, we will not cover the many edible wild plants and animals that are available in North America.

EDIBLE WILD PLANTS

For those who think they cannot go for three days without eating three meals a day, I would suggest they read and study the many survival books and other books which describe and show detail photos of the approximately two thousand edible wild plants and seven hundred toxic wild plants found in North America. Distinguishing one from the other requires a lot of field experience during all four seasons. A book like this cannot scratch the surface on this subject. A book that does is the *Scouting Guide to Foraging*, also available from Skyhorse Publishing.

WILD PLANT EDIBILITY TEST

If for some reason you are in a situation where there are wild plants you think you must eat but don't know which ones are edible, the US Air Force Survival School Edibility Test may be of some help:
1. Never use mushrooms or fungi.
2. Poisonous plant life means all parts, including flowers, can be toxic. Use caution with plants having these characteristics:
    »   Milky or discolored sap
    »   Spines or fine hairs
    »   Bitter or soapy taste

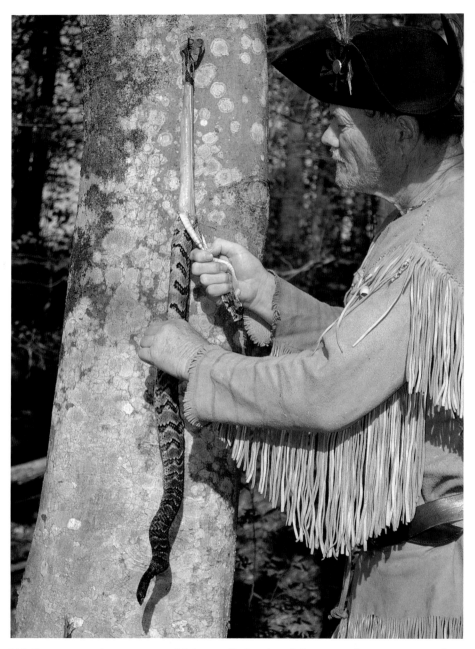

While mountain men could live off the land for months at a time, few among us today have those skills. Since the majority of lost or stranded people are found within seventy-two hours, starvation is not a likely threat.

THE SCOUT'S GUIDE TO WILDERNESS SURVIVAL AND FIRST AID

- » Beans or bulbs
- » White or red berries
- » Shiny leaves
- » Umbrella flowers

3. Take a small mouthful and chew it. Wait five minutes for any effects such as burning, stinging, or numbing.
4. If there is none, swallow and wait eight hours for any effects such as diarrhea, cramps, pain, numbing, or vomiting.
5. If there is none, repeat the process, using a handful of the plant, and wait another eight hours for ill effects.
6. If none, the plant is considered safe to eat.

Keep in mind that any new or strange food should be eaten with restraint until the body system has become accustomed to it. Also, don't expect wild plants to taste good. Many don't, and others are almost tasteless. It takes some adjusting to get your stomach to accept a diet of wild plants.

Some other things you need to know about wild plants:

1. Plants you see animals eating may be toxic to man. Deer love poison ivy, for example.
2. Plants that you may eat in one stage may not be edible in other stages of growth. Pokeweed is a good example of this.
3. Some parts of plants may be edible while others may not be. Wild plum is an example of this.

EDIBLE WILD ANIMALS

If the survivor really must resort to wild foods in order not to starve to death, then wild animals may be a better choice than wild plants, if he or she has hunting or trapping skills. North America has a good population of wild animals, both large and small, that are edible. The trick is that you first must get them before you can cook them. Even the Lewis and Clark Expedition members, at one point, almost starved to death due to not killing any game to eat, and had to depend upon roots.

Depending upon the time of year and where you are geographically, there is some form of animal that you can eat if you can get it. Insects and small aquatic animals may be the easiest to gather and highest in protein, but what if it is winter? There may be an abundance of larger animals, but if you lack the skills necessary to kill the animals, you can go hungry. And remember, animals are often hard to find even by the most skilled hunters. Provided you can kill them, wild animals are a good source of food and may be cooked over the survival fire with ease. Just don't expect them to taste like home cooking.

Survival food is not an important need for the short term. Shelter and signaling are. Accept the fact that the last thing you should concern yourself with is the procurement of food. If you have filed a trip plan with a responsible person and you stopped just as soon as you knew you were in trouble, you will be rescued long before your hunger pains become serious. Think of this experience as the beginning of that diet you have been considering.

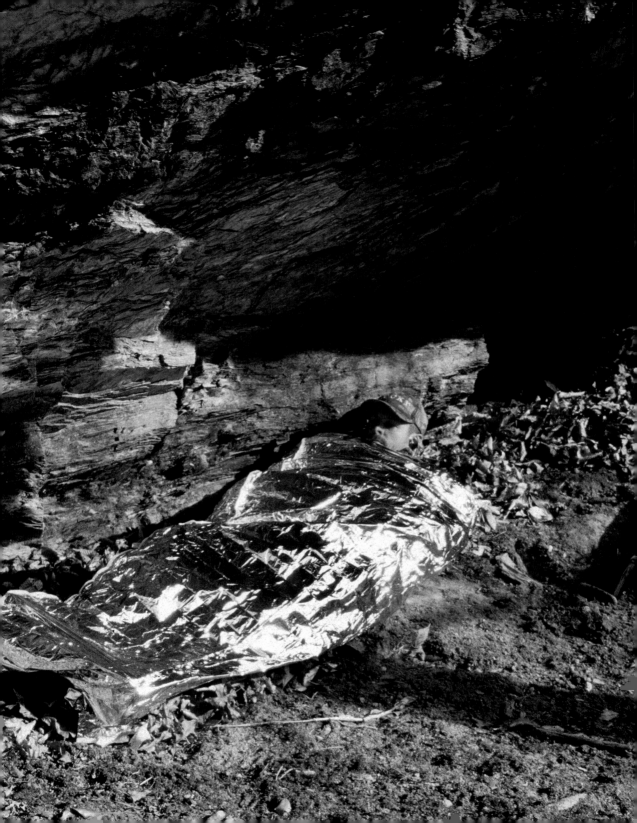

12

IMPORTANCE OF GETTING SLEEP

Sleeping warm and comfortably cannot be emphasized enough in the survival emergency. You need a lot of energy for the tasks at hand, and the mind needs to be sharper than during your normal day-to-day life, as the decisions you make will determine your well-being and the outcome of your situation.

If you have a tube tent and emergency sleeping bag in your survival kit and set up the tube tent so that you can get into the bag before you get wet, then chances are good you will sleep warm. How well you clean the tube tent site will determine how comfortably you sleep. Remember you do not have an air mattress or anything else thick between you and the ground. A few minutes spent removing stones, sticks, and other debris and laying down a bed of dry leaves can make the difference between an uncomfortable night and a comfortable one.

But what about a night spent without the aid of a tube tent or emergency sleeping bag? In this case there are several options, depending upon the terrain where you determine to camp. The first rule is to get into a shelter of some type that can give you protection from the rain, snow, or wind; if the shelter is conducive to having a fire, so much the better. Your chances of actually getting some sleep improve when you can stay warm. Be sure to gather three times as much wood as you think you will need, as it will probably take it to keep the fire going all night. It is difficult to keep the body warm or to get enough sleep when you must make two or three trips out into the cold darkness to gather up fuel wood.

The ideal sleeping shelter, aside from the tube tent/emergency sleeping bag combination, is the well-made lean-to with its back to the wind and a reflector fire directing heat into the shelter. Using a sheet of aluminum foil, a wall of green limbs, rocks, and so on as a reflector, the all-night fire can keep a lean-to reasonably warm throughout the night as long as there is enough fuel wood. As the fire dies down, you simply toss on enough wood to keep it going another few hours.

When rain or snow is not a threat, a reflector fire directing heat to a large rock or dirt bank, blocking the wind, can make a nice place to sleep. The heat is reflected to the rock or bank and back onto you while you sleep. You have heat from two sides.

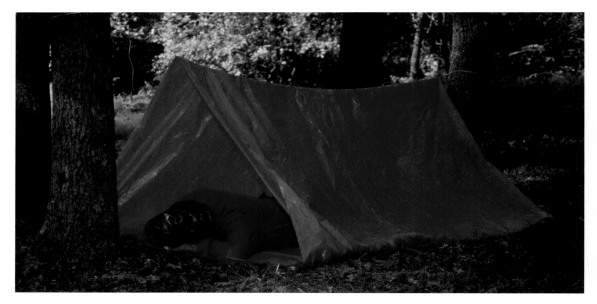

Getting a restful night's sleep is essential to keeping the mind sharp. This will help you make good decisions towards being rescued.

You can build a fire on the spot you plan on sleeping and let it warm up the earth for a few hours, then rack the fire away to a new spot and sleep on the warm earth. If you have a means of digging, you can dig a shallow hole where your body is going to lie, shovel in a bed of hot ashes, and cover it with a layer of soil. Make sure to cover all the ashes and give it a "try and see" test. If you have enough cover soil on, you will have a bed that's not too hot or too cold. This is an energy-consuming means of having a warm bed.

Some experienced backwoodsmen heat a number of flat rocks and place them on the ground. Next they place a thick layer of precut evergreen boughs over the rocks and sleep on them. Again, this type of warm sleeping requires a lot of energy and experience.

If you don't have an emergency bag, sleeping bag, or blanket, you can use dry dead grass, leaves, or evergreen boughs to give you some protection from the cold. Remember that insulation is dead air space and anything that will create dead air space will help keep you warm. The rainsuit can offer a lot of warmth when sleeping due to its ability to stop the wind. By stuffing dead, dry grass or leaves inside the rainsuit, you can also make a makeshift sleeping bag. Be resourceful.

Here are some tips for getting a good night's sleep:

- Take the time to make the bed site as level and soft as possible.
- Be sure to use every windbreak available.
- Gather three times as much firewood as you will think you need.
- Eat sweets just before bedtime, if you have them, to boost your metabolism.

- Do not lie awake the first night expecting searchers every minute. You will hear them if they get close and you will need to be rested the next day.
- At night, due to your situation, your senses will be acutely aware and you will hear every noise. Remember there is nothing out there that will hurt you.
- When sleeping with your clothing on, keep everything loose, including boots. The better circulation you have, the warmer you will sleep. This also permits moisture to evaporate.

You can bet that even in the best of circumstances you are not going to sleep in the survival camp as well as you do at home, but with a little care you can get some sleep and that rest is most important to getting found.

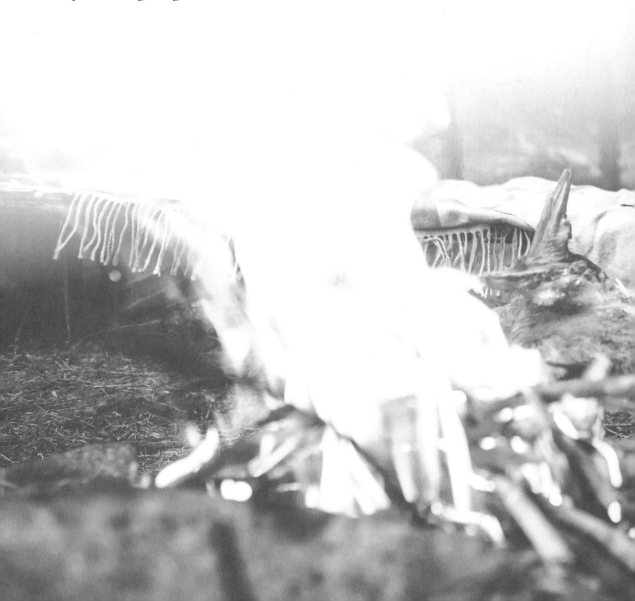

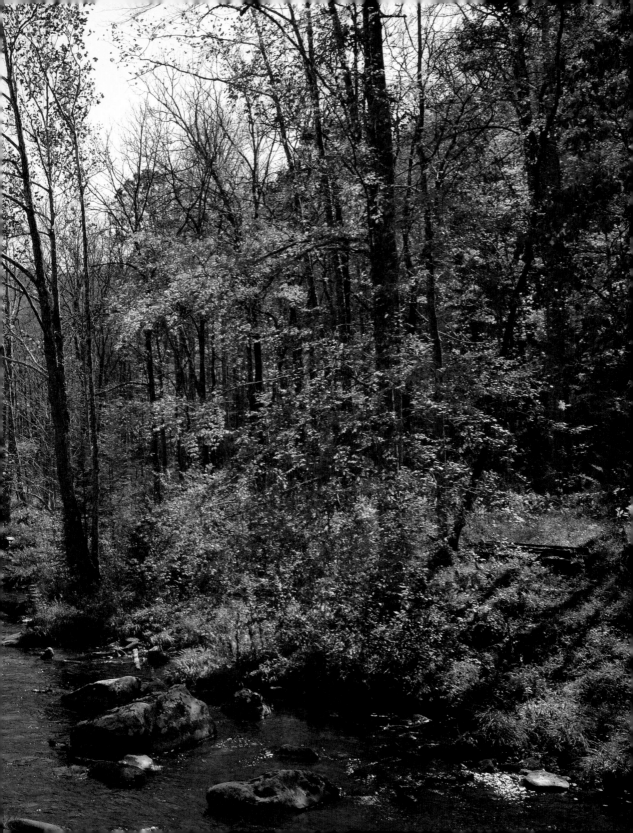

13

DEALING WITH INSECTS AND SPIDERS

Few things can ruin an outdoor adventure faster than hordes of mosquitoes and/or blackflies. In large numbers, they have been known to bring armies to a halt, stampede animals, and turn countless camping trips into horror stories. In a stranded or lost emergency, they can become very dangerous. Even in cold areas, a sudden warm snap can bring out the pests in numbers.

Of the more than 1,600 varieties of mosquitoes, 120 are found in the North America. Many of these are known to transmit such diseases as West Nile virus, encephalitis, and dengue fever. Just their bites alone, in high numbers, are very dangerous.

Nuisance bugs are a part of many outdoor trips, but with a little planning, and preventive measures, they will not spoil the fun of the trip. Here are some ways to keep your encounters with these "critters" to a minimum.

- Cool weather sends these insects away, so when practical, plan your outdoor trip in cold weather.
- Call ahead and find out if the area you are going into has any potential nuisance bug activity during the time you will be visiting. If so, find out what and plan preventive measures.
- If you are going into an area with a pest you have no experience with, take the time to know how to avoid or repel them. Say you are from the North and have never encountered fire ants. Go to a little trouble and learn how to recognize their mounds. If you are forced to wade in flooded areas, know that fire ants survive floods by forming a ball as large as a basketball and floating to dry ground. You don't want your fishing waders to be the dry spot they rub up against.

- Black widow and brown recluse spiders usually stay hidden, so when in their areas, be safe by shaking out your clothing and footwear before putting them on and by not putting your hands into secluded areas when you're out in the woods. When using outhouses, always check under the seat, a favorite home range for black widows.
- Chiggers thrive in heavy vegetation, so during warm weather, don't get into thick vines and leaves. This helps avoid ticks as well.
- For repelling ticks, chiggers, deer flies, and horse flies, spray your clothing with permethrin-based repellent. Apply a Deet-based repellent to your exposed skin. Deet-based repellents last only a few hours, whereas permethrin-based repellents applied only to clothing last for several days. Be sure to read the labels of each product and follow the instructions.
- Stinging insects such as hornets, bees, and yellow jackets usually only require that you give their nests a wide berth. In the fall, bees and yellow jackets will often come to your picnic lunch and you will have to use more caution at that time.
- Mosquitoes and blackflies can be kept at bay by using a Deet-based repellent or by using the very effective Thermacell repellent appliance. Keeping exposed skin to a minimum, such as using a head net and taping sleeves and pant legs closed, also helps keeps the blood-sucking damage to a minimum.

Insects are a valuable part of the outdoor world, and with a little knowledge, planning, and repellent, we can share the outdoors with them without suffering.

To deal with these flying pests, we need to know more about them.

MOSQUITOES

Mosquitoes mature in standing water. It is the female mosquito that causes us grief, as she needs a high-protein meal before she is able to lay her eggs. Physiological restrictions make it impossible for her to eat anything which is not in liquid form, and the handiest liquid, high-protein meal available to her is blood. The male mosquito is a vegetarian and feeds on plant and fruit nectar.

Sensors, which are attracted to warm, moist animals, help the female mosquito locate a meal. The generally accepted theory in the scientific community is that the mosquito finds its victim by identifying and following carbon dioxide and lactic acid in the air. Lactic acid is produced by muscle movement, and carbon dioxide is given off when we breathe.

Once she finds a victim, she penetrates the victim's skin with a hollow, flexible snout, called a proboscis, and feeds. The itch and local swelling around the "bite" is an allergic reaction to the mosquito's saliva, which contains an anticoagulant to facilitate the flow of blood.

BLACKFLIES

For those who have been bitten by blackflies, the bite is a form of torture. These small, humpbacked flies have few equals when it comes to inflicting pain. Of over three hundred varieties of blackflies in the world, North America has been cursed with at least fifty of them.

Unlike the mosquito, the blackfly thrives in running water. Rapidly flowing streams are preferred breeding places. Once able to fly, the female, which feeds by day, is ready for a meal in order to carry out its task of reproduction.

Like the mosquito, the blackfly is found over much of North America, but its largest concentrations are in the woodlands of Canada and the northern reaches of the United States. This insect is abundant throughout late spring and summer, with May and June being the worst months in many areas.

The vicious bite of the blackfly is caused by broad blades found in the mouth parts. These blades make relatively large wounds, which continue to bleed after the fly has fed and gone. The bite often goes unnoticed until a trickle of blood is felt or seen. Blackfly saliva may be toxic, causing pain and itching and sometimes nervous and intestinal disorders.

Not as much is known about the blackfly as about the mosquito, so we can't say what actually draws this insect to its target. But it is thought that the female blackfly detects the carbon dioxide given off by the skin and then follows the convection currents of warm moist air that the host produces.

Repellent Use

Anyone who is going into the backcountry should always carry a good supply of chemical insect repellent, even if the trip is to be a short one. A repellent should always be included in a survival kit. Repellents are the most effective deterrent. They work by confusing the insect and discouraging it from feeding on the victim.

The percentage of DEET in an insect repellent can determine how long the product will give you protection. If the insect repellent you purchase has 10 to 15 percent DEET, you can expect approximately four hours of protection; from 20 to 50 percent, approximately six hours; 50 to 75 percent, approximately eight hours; and 75 to 100 percent, a full day of protection. This varies from person to person, but it is a good rule of thumb to start with.

People who spend a lot of time in the outdoors today are blessed with a number of excellent insect repellents to choose from. I carry BugX repellent single-use towelettes in my survival kit. They take up little space and work well.

When using any of these chemical repellents, you should follow some simple guidelines:

1. Read all label directions carefully.
2. When using aerosol repellents, always keep the spray opening aimed away from your face, and avoid spraying while close to fire.

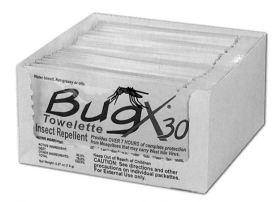

Towelettes, such as the BugX brand insect repellent, are an excellent way to pack in enough protection to last several days.

3. For the best protection, repellent should be applied to all exposed skin except eyes, lips, and open cuts.
4. Avoid repellent contact with outdoor equipment and clothing made of Spandex, rayon, acrylics, or plastics. It can dissolve monofilament fishing line, and plastic lenses in glasses.
5. Reapply repellent after swimming or perspiring heavily, since water or perspiration will weaken a repellent's effectiveness.

Repellents alone will not give you total protection from mosquitoes and blackflies in areas of heavy infestations. A head net may be well worth the bother at certain times.

In bug country, you should always wear a long-sleeved shirt and pants. Apply a repellent containing an appropriate percentage of DEET to the clothing as well as to your exposed skin. To keep the pests from invading the openings of your clothing, use rubber bands or short lengths of cord to tie down your shirt sleeves and pants legs.

When using a repellent, the trick is to apply enough to get complete coverage. According to experts, it takes approximately five seconds of spray time to cover the wrist to the elbow. Most people try to do it in less than one second.

For tick and chigger control, spray clothing and gear, such as day packs, with permethrin. It kills these insects as well as mosquitoes on contact. Be sure to follow the instructions on the label.

In a survival situation during warm weather, pick a campsite with insect control in mind. Stay away from pools of stagnant water. Pick sites that are on high breezy points or at least in the open where you can take advantage of any breeze that may help keep the insects away.

When there is No Repellent

There are often occasions where the lost or stranded person either has run out of repellent or has none and the flying pests are out in vast numbers. When this happens, the first thing to do is to cover up all exposed skin areas. Tuck trouser legs down into boots. Button sleeves tight around the wrist. Pull up shirt and coat collars to protect the neck. Put on a hat and gloves. In short, give the biting critters as small a target as possible.

Next, build a smoky fire near your shelter; at a time like this, the smokier the better. Lie down and put your face near the ground to keep your eyes and nose as free of the smoke as possible. While this may be irritating, it is better than being fed on by flying pests. In severe conditions, build two fires and sit in the middle. There is no good substitute for carrying insect repellent in your survival kit.

TICKS

While ticks are a potential long-term health threat with diseases such as Lyme disease or Rocky Mountain spotted fever, they do not pose the immediate threat that large numbers of flying pests do. Ticks should be avoided, and when found on the body, removed.

The best prevention is to conduct a full-body tick check using a hand-held mirror—your signal mirror may work—to view all parts of your body upon return from tick-infested areas. Look for ticks under the arms, in and around the ears, inside the belly button, behind the knees, between the legs, around the waist, and especially in hair. Examine gear and pets. Ticks can ride into the survival camp on clothing and pets, then attach to a person later, so carefully examine pets, coats, and daypacks.

The recommended way to remove an embedded tick is discussed in Chapter 29, "Infectious Diseases."

SPIDERS

Spiders seem to scare almost as many people as snakes do. However, most spiders are harmless to man. In fact, about seven people die from spider bites in North America in any given year. The two North American spiders that can be deadly are the black widow and the brown recluse. (See treatment for these bites in Chapter 26 of the First Aid section.)

Black Widow Spider

The female black widow is far more of a toxic hazard than the male She has a shiny black body, approximately 0.6 inch long, and usually has a red hourglass-shaped mark on the underside of her globular abdomen On some, the hourglass marking is replaced with several triangles or spots or an irregular longitudinal blotch She has slim black legs with a span of 1.5 inches. The less toxic male is considerably smaller than the female and usually is a patterned brown color.

The black widow is found throughout North America except in northern Canada and in Alaska. Most reported human fatalities have occurred in the southeastern states.

The black widow is generally found in its irregular-shaped web near the ground. Common web sites are under stones, loose bark, or water faucets, or in woodpiles, rodent burrows, garages, storage buildings, outhouses,

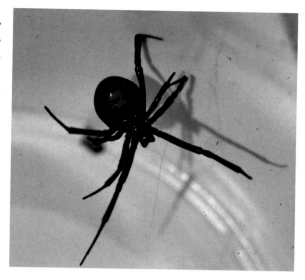

The black widow spider is slow to bite and prefers no contact with man.

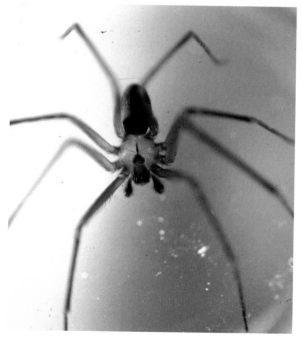

The brown recluse spider can be identified by the violin-shaped markings on head and thorax.

and barns. Most human bites occur when the spider is inadvertently trapped against part of the body or when the web is accidentally touched.

Man is seldom bitten by the black widow, but when it happens, the bite can be serious.

Brown Recluse Spider

The brown recluse is a medium-sized spider with leg span from 0.8 to 1.6 inches and a color range from yellow-tan to dark brown. The most distinguishing characteristics are its six eyes (most spiders have eight eyes) arranged a semicircle of three pairs on top of the head, and a violin-shaped marking extending from the area of the eyes to the abdomen.

Brown recluse spiders are found throughout much of the United States. They will readily establish populations inside parts of a building that are generally dry, littered, and undisturbed for long periods. The spiders can also be found outside the protected areas under rocks and loose bark. Members of this species are nonaggressive and normally attempt to escape whenever they are threatened. Thus, most instances of bites occur when the spider is inadvertently trapped, such as when the victim puts on clothing in which the spider is hiding, steps barefoot on a wandering spider at night, or cleans storage areas where the spider resides.

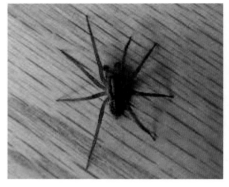

Hobo Spider

The hobo spider is found in southern British Columbia, Washington, Oregon, Idaho, western Montana, western Wyoming, and northern Utah.

A hobo spider.

Hobo spiders frequent areas such as log or timber piles, rock piles, holes in logs/trees, or where tall grass meets crevices in soil where they can make their characteristic funnel webs. The webs are funnel shaped, narrow at the bottom, wide at the top. The spider waits in the small hole at the bottom of the funnel for prey to make contact with the web. When it senses a vibration it will emerge from the hole to envenomate its prey.

The hobo spider has a brown front body region where the legs are attached with darker brown markings and brown legs. The abdomen has a distinctive pattern of yellow markings on a gray background, although this pattern can be difficult to discern without the aid of a microscope or hand lens. The pattern is generally more distinctive in immature specimens. Unlike many other similar-looking spiders, hobo spiders do not have dark bands on their legs. Spiders with such banding are not hobo spiders.

Mature female hobo spiders are 3/8 to 5/8-inches long, and male hobo spiders are 9/32 to 9/16 inches in body length. Males have enlarged pedipalps located near the mouth, resembling short legs.

Bites from some other spiders can be painful and can lead to infections, but they do not pose the hazard of toxins associated with the brown recluse, hobo, or black widow.

14

POTENTIAL DANGERS

Anyone going into wilderness areas should be aware of the potential dangers that exist. I say potential, as many adventurers spend a lifetime of going into the wilderness areas of North America and never encounter any of these threats. Yet every year scores of outings are ruined due to one or more of these dangers occurring, sometimes with fatal consequences. It is better to have thought out these dangers ahead of time and know how to handle them than it is to go on an outing without a clue.

Also, some of these dangers are the reasons some people stay out of the wilderness. Perhaps if they knew more about these dangers and how to avoid them, they would be ready to face the outdoors with a positive attitude and enjoy their outings.

SNAKES

In my survival seminars I can mention that automobile accidents kill some 40,000 Americans each year, and no one becomes troubled. I can tell the students that lightning kills around thirty Americans annually, and no one raises an eyebrow. But the mention of venomous snakes, which kill fewer than a dozen Americans annually, sends everyone squirming or climbing up on chairs. For some unknown reason, snakes scare the otherwise most fearless among us. Basically, this is an excessive fear—a phobia.

Venomous snakes are found in all the states with the exception of Maine, Alaska, and Hawaii. Canada has rattlesnakes in southern British Columbia, Alberta, Saskatchewan, and Ontario. North America's venomous snakes include two species of coral snakes, four subspecies of copperhead, three subspecies of cottonmouth, and sixteen species of rattlesnakes.

Rattlesnakes are known from elevations up to eleven thousand feet in the southern Sierra Nevada of California, to about eight thousand feet on dry, rocky slopes in Montana, and to the tops of the highest mountains in the Appalachians. In spite of this, venomous snakes are rare in high mountains of the West, in northern evergreen forests, and in heavily farmed or urban industrial areas.

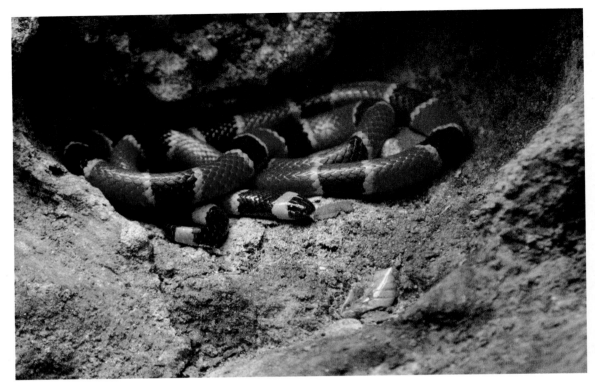

A coral snake; note red bands touch yellow bands.

Surprisingly, some species survive well in suburban areas, especially in the southern states. Areas with unusually large populations of venomous snakes include parts of the Great Plains (rattlesnakes), the lower Mississippi Valley and Gulf Coast (rattlesnakes and cottonmouths), and the southern Appalachians (rattlesnakes and copperheads).

Snakebite is by no means rare in the southern and western United States. Incidence is highest in children from five to fifteen years old, and most bites are sustained close to home. Many bites result from deliberate handling of venomous snakes. (Treatment for venomous snakebite is found in Chapter 26 of the First Aid section.)

Try to learn to identify poisonous snakes and where they are found.

Coral Snake

This pretty but deadly snake is found in the southern United States from the lowlands of North Carolina to the southwestern states. Coral snakes are usually from twenty to thirty inches long. The coral snake has colored rings completely encircling the body. The colors are red, yellow, and black. A positive identification of the coral snake is that the red ring touches the yellow ring. Coral snakes are usually secretive and hide in leaves, logs, stumps, and debris.

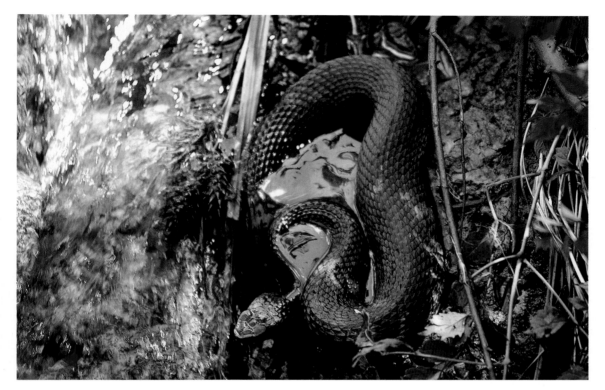

The cottonmouth can be aggressive and giving them a lot of space is the best way to deal with them.

Cottonmouth (Water Moccasin)

The color pattern of the cottonmouth, often called water moccasin, is dull and inconspicuous: dark-brown bars on a somewhat lighter background. Many cottonmouths look either dirty brown or uniform black. I have seen some that were difficult to identify because of variance in their color patterns. The most positive identification is the elliptical, cat-like pupil of the eye, but you don't want to be that close in order to identify it. The cottonmouths get their name from their habit of threatening an intruder with open mouth, revealing a cotton-white interior. Although some individual cottonmouths exceed five feet in length, most are from three to four feet long.

The cottonmouth range is much smaller than most people believe. Generally, their range runs south of a line from south-central Texas up through the Mississippi River Basin in Missouri, down along the Tennessee River Basin, and up the East Coast where the elevation is below eight hundred feet. More often than not, supposed cottonmouths turn out to be voracious water snakes that belong to the *Nerodia* species. These snakes are aggressive, and some do resemble the cottonmouth, but they are not venomous.

Though the cottonmouth is much scarcer than many believe, when you encounter one, avoid it. It is curious and is no coward. The cottonmouth is slow to retreat. Many times I have seen one stand its ground when escape would have been easy.

The best prevention against a cottonmouth bite is precaution. When you are in cottonmouth territory, keep your eyes open and always watch where you place your feet and hands. When you travel in a boat, watch overhanging limbs, stumps, logs, and the base of trees. Cottonmouths like to sun themselves, as other snakes do. Several times I have almost grabbed a snake by reaching around a tree to tie up a boat. Look before you put your hands anywhere.

Another place you are likely to encounter a cottonmouth is on the end of your fish stringer. There is no more sobering experience than to pull up a stringer of fish and find a big cottonmouth attached, swallowing one of the fish. That hazard is one reason southern fishermen have an ice chest or live-well in which to keep their catches.

Copperhead

The copperhead's back is pinkish-buff, russet, or orange-brown with dark brown to reddish cross bands; the belly is pinkish-white with large dark spots, or mottling; the top of the head is yellowish to coppery red; the sides are paler; and the end of the tail is yellow in young snakes, black to dark greenish or brown in adults. The cross band is narrow in the center of the back and wide on the sides in eastern specimens, only slightly narrowed in western ones. The copperhead being a pit viper, the pupil of the eye is elliptical. The average length is two to three feet; maximum, slightly over four feet.

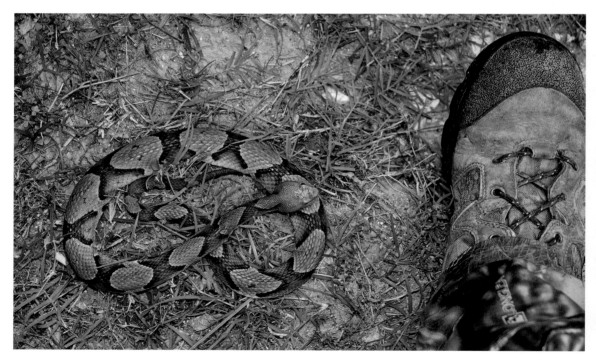

The copperhead is usually slow to anger and well camouflaged for the woodland floor in which he is found.

The copperhead is found in the eastern US (Massachusetts to Kansas, south to the Gulf Coast, westward into Trans-Pecos, Texas), and the southern plains. It frequents wooded, hilly country in the North and West, lowlands in the South, and is sometimes plentiful in well-populated areas. Nocturnal in warm weather, it is diurnal in cool weather. In rocky country, it frequently hibernates in rocky dens with rattlesnakes and various nonpoisonous species.

When encountered, the copperhead usually remains coiled and quiet unless closely approached or touched. It vibrates its tail when angry, and often seems reluctant to strike, although some individuals are very irritable.

Copperheads account for the great majority of snakebites received in the eastern United States, exclusive of Florida and the Mississippi Delta. However, fatalities from these bites are almost unknown.

Rattlesnake

Of the poisonous snakes found in North America, the rattlesnake is perhaps the easiest to identify, because of the jointed rattle found at the tip of the tail. However, this is not always the case because the rattle can be broken off. The pupil of the rattlesnake's eye is vertically elliptical, as is that of the copperhead and cottonmouth.

The rattlesnake is found throughout the United States except in Maine, Alaska, and Hawaii. It is also found in southern British Columbia, Alberta, Saskatchewan, and Ontario in Canada.

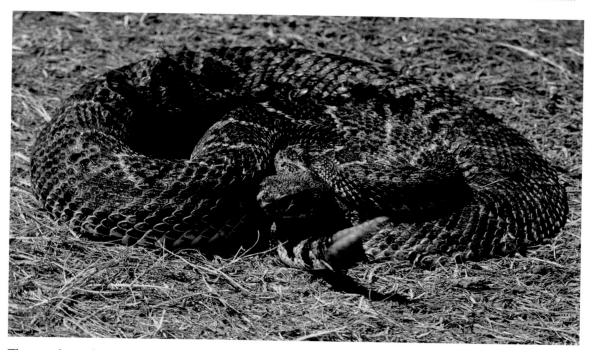

The rattlesnake likes to lay up in the cool shade during the day and venture out to feed at night, a good reason to stay put in your survival camp at night.

Here are some don'ts to follow when in snake country:

1. Don't put your hands or feet in places you cannot look, and don't put them in places without first looking.
2. Don't turn or lift a rock or fallen tree with your hands. Move it with a stick or with your foot if your ankle and leg are properly protected.
3. Don't disturb snakes.
4. Don't put your sleeping bag near rock piles or rubbish piles or near the entrance to a cave.
5. Don't sit down without first looking around carefully.
6. Don't gather firewood after dark.
7. Don't step over a log if the other side is not visible. Step on it first.
8. Don't enter snake-infested areas without adequate protective clothing.
9. Don't handle freshly killed venomous snakes.
10. Don't crawl under a fence in high grass or in an uncleared area.
11. Don't go out of your way to kill a poisonous snake unless you need the meat to survive. Thousands of people are bitten by snakes each year merely because they try to kill them without knowing anything of their habits or habitats.
12. Don't panic!

Snakes are probably one of the most overrated fears in the outdoors, and the odds are fairly high that you will never see one or, greater yet, get bitten. However, the potential does exist and some commonsense precaution should be taken. Remember, snakes do not want any more contact with you than you with them.

LIGHTNING

Lightning is one of nature's forces that I respect most. I have been the victim of an indirect strike of lightning twice and on numerous occasions I have seen the destruction it can cause in a second.

Here is just one example of how lightning can become a danger within seconds. It was a perfect day as a scoutmaster led his scout troop into the backcountry of the Great Smoky Mountains National Park. Mid-afternoon found the backpackers in a low valley as they walked toward Molly Ridge. Suddenly the bright sky turned dark and a hard rainstorm blew in from behind a tall mountain. Without any warning there was a bright flash and resounding crack as a lightning bolt, the only one of the storm, found its way from the storm cloud to the earth. The lightning forked on its way and hit five trees within a one-hundred-yard diameter. None of the trees were particularly tall as compared to the surrounding trees. From one of the trees, the lightning bolt arced ten feet and struck the scoutmaster's metal pack frame. Traveling down the frame, melting the aluminum as it went, the lightning entered his body at the lower end of the frame where it touches the small of the back. From there it traveled down his legs, shredding his pants into specks of cloth, twisted both ankles and ripped off both boots, and blew off the little toe on the foot that was not touching the ground. Leaving his body, the bolt continued downhill, plowing

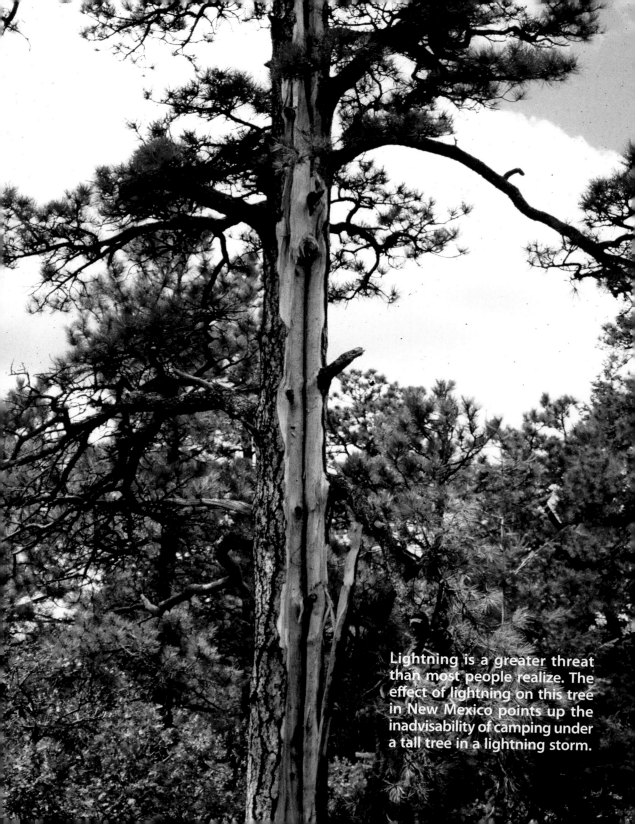

Lightning is a greater threat than most people realize. The effect of lightning on this tree in New Mexico points up the inadvisability of camping under a tall tree in a lightning storm.

a ditch as it went. Four other troop members, some one hundred yards away, were knocked down and stunned by the same bolt.

The scoutmaster fell to the ground alive but severely hurt.

The rest of the story is a credit to leadership, training, and courage. Due to the efforts of his scouts and the park rangers, the scoutmaster was in the hospital late that night. It was twenty-six days before he could go home, and he carries the scars today to prove that lightning can be a deadly killer even in low valleys.

Each year in the US lightning, on average, kills thirty people. It is also the greatest single cause of forest fires in the western US, starting over 7,500 fires each year.

Lightning is not only a killer of man, but it also kills many animals each year, both wild and domestic. As I was researching this book, lightning struck a tree in the middle of a pasture near where I live and killed fifty head of beef cattle, weighing about eight hundred pounds each, who were standing under the tree. There are many reports by wildlife biologists each year of deer and elk being killed by lightning.

The coasts of the US over the years have had a high number of lightning fatalities, with a higher-than-average incidence of lightning fatalities and property damage along the Mississippi, Ohio, and Hudson rivers and their drainage basins. The Rocky Mountains are also hard hit by lightning. However, all areas of North America can experience sudden storms with lightning, so the rule for anyone outdoors is to always keep an eye on the weather.

From studies drawn from years of case histories provided by the National Weather Service, the National Climatic Center, and other agencies, it has been possible to draw up a list of useful safety rules for surviving lightning.

First, of course, is to get the latest weather forecast before setting forth to go outside, or before embarking on a recreational outing. If there is a chance of thunderstorm, take a cell phone with a weather app along to get occasional updates, and be ready to seek shelter if a severe thunderstorm watch or warning is announced. The more severe the thunderstorm, the greater the intensity and frequency of lightning strokes.

You don't need an official warning to tell you that a thunderstorm is coming. In almost all cases you can see the towering thunder-head and occasional flashes of lightning at least half an hour in advance. Usually this is ample time to find shelter or take precautions.

When a thunderstorm threatens, all lightning experts agree that the single most important thing you can do is to get inside a home or a large building, or inside an all-metal automobile.

Outdoor recreationists frequently overlook the fact that their automobile is an excellent lightning shelter. This is so because the metal of the car conducts the lightning current around the people safely tucked inside. Many believe the rubber tires insulate the car from a lightning strike. Some of these people also believe it is safe in the bed of a pickup truck or on the seat of a tractor because of the tires, but they are wrong. Lightning, after traveling miles through insulating air, has no trouble flashing across the tires. A car struck by lightning will almost always be found with the occupants unhurt but with the tires blown or aflame.

Other rules to follow:

- Do not stand underneath a natural lightning rod such as a large tree in an open area.
- Avoid projecting above the surrounding landscape, as you would do if you were standing on a hilltop, in an open field, on the beach, paddling a canoe in a lake, or fishing from a small boat.
- Get out of and away from open water. (If you're swimming, lightning current from a nearby stroke can flow through the water to you.)
- Get away from metal objects such as an ATV, barbecue, or wire fence.
- Fishing rods of all materials can become lightning rods if elevated above the hull of a boat or canoe. Lower rods and lay in bottom of craft at the first sight of lightning.
- Avoid standing in small isolated sheds or other small structures in open areas.
- In a forest, seek shelter in a low area under a thick growth of small trees. In open areas, go to a low place such as a ravine or valley.
- Groups of persons in exposed situations, such as hikers or mountain climbers, should spread out—staying several yards apart—so that if lightning strikes nearby, the smallest number will be affected.
- Stay away from water, wet items such as ropes, and metal objects such as fences and poles. Water and metal do not attract lightning but they are excellent conductors of electricity. The current from a lightning flash will easily travel for long distances.

Keeping an eye on the weather and keeping in touch with a current weather report is always the best way to prepare for an electrical storm.

FLASH FLOODING

The transformation of a tranquil river or scenic dry canyon into a destructive flood occurs hundreds of times each year. No area of North America is completely free from the threat of flash flooding.

Take Colorado as an example. Flash floods are no strangers to Colorado outdoorsmen. Since the year 1900, nearly three hundred people have been killed in flash floods across that one state.

In terms of lives lost, the worst flash flood occurred on July 31, 1976 in the Big Thompson Canyon between Estes Park and Loveland, Colorado. A nearly stationary storm produced around twelve inches of rain within four hours, claiming 144 lives, mostly campers.

Flash floods are a fact of life—and death—along the rivers and streambeds and arroyos of North America. They result from rains and/or melting snow filling natural and man-made drainage systems to overflowing with raging water and its deadly cargo of uprooted trees, smashed structures, boulders, mud, and other debris.

The US Department of Commerce's National Oceanic and Atmospheric Administration (NOAA) and its National Weather Service have taken steps to improve the technology and content of our flood warning system and to increase the time available for people to take emergency measures to protect life and property. With flash floods, time is so short and the possibility of tragedy so great that individuals in many areas must also utilize local preparedness plans to help themselves. If you understand the danger of flash flooding and know what immediate action to take, you can save your life.

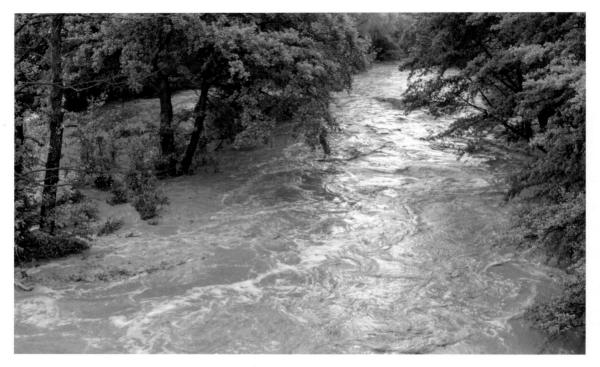

The National Weather Service has two flash flood alerts which they issue. These alerts should be given everyone's attention in the specific area.

Flash Flood Watch. Heavy rains may result in flash flooding in the specified area. Be alert and prepared for the possibility of a flood emergency that will require immediate action. Have a plan to move to higher ground quickly.

Flash Flood Warning. Flash flooding is occurring or is imminent in the specified areas. Move to safe ground immediately.

Before the flood, know the elevation of your location in relation to nearby streams and other waterways, and make advance plans of what you will do and where you will go in a flash flood emergency.

When a flash flood watch is issued for your area:

- Listen to area radio stations on a battery-operated weather radio or watch weather apps on your cell phone for possible flash flood warnings and reports of flooding in progress from the National Weather Service and public safety agencies.
- Be prepared to move out of danger's way at a moment's notice.
- If you are on a road, watch for flooding at highway dips, bridges, and low areas.
- Watch for signs (thunder, lightning) of distant heavy rainfall. It may not be raining where you are, but it may be pouring down at the upper end of the watershed you are in and a wall of water may be racing toward you.

When a flash flood warning is issued for your area:

- Act quickly to save yourself and those who depend on you. You may have only seconds.
- Do not attempt to cross a flowing stream on foot where water is above your knees. Even then, use a wading pole to keep your balance.
- If you are driving, don't try to ford dips of unknown depth. If your vehicle stalls, abandon it immediately and seek higher ground, as rapidly rising water may sweep the vehicle and its occupants away. Many deaths have been caused by attempts to move stalled vehicles. Remember that it takes little over one foot of water to carry most cars and trucks away. Turn around, don't drown.
- Be especially cautious at night, when it is harder to recognize flood dangers.

After the flash flood watch or warning has been cancelled, stay tuned to radio or weather apps for follow-up information. Flash flooding may have ended, but general flooding may come later in headwater streams and major rivers. Remember, any heavy rain can cause locally destructive flash flooding. Any time you are in the backcountry and it is raining, think flash floods.

Heavy rainfall, even for short periods, may be followed by flash flooding in mountainous or hilly areas. When you go into remote areas, follow these suggestions:

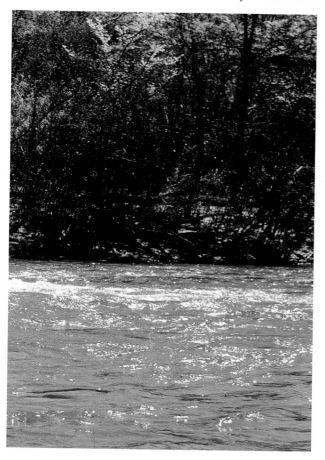

- Stay away from natural streambeds, arroyos, and other drainage channels during and after rainstorms. Water runs off the higher elevations very rapidly.
- Never camp on low ground. A flash flood can catch you while you sleep.
- Use your topo maps. Know where you are and whether you are on low ground.
- Remember, you don't have to be at the bottom of a hill to be a target for flash flood dangers.
- Know where the high ground is and how to get there.
- Stay out of flooded areas.

- Keep alert to signs of wet weather, either rain where you are or signs of rain, including thunder and nearby lightning.
- Keep as informed as you can.

If you are out of range of broadcast/cell phone information, be sure to watch for these indicators of flash flooding:

- Storms nearby.
- Increase in the speed of river flow.
- Rapid rise in river level.

Be prepared to move to safety quickly.

FALLS

Falls are one of the most common accidents that happen in the wilderness each year. An attractive waterfall, cliff, log over a rushing stream, muddy slope, or cave can all be the attraction that can cause a serious fall and resulting injuries that lead to a stranding and a survival situation. People who become lost often panic and start running, and that can lead to serious falls. Falls and the resulting injuries or death are one of the most frequent reasons for search and rescue efforts.

A book could be written about how to prevent falls in the wilderness, but here are just a few of the precautions to take:

- Falls can result in serious injuries or death and put you in a survival situation fast. Take fall prevention seriously. Don't take chances.
- Watch where you are walking. Wet leaves, tree roots, mud, ice, snow, wet grass, and wet logs have all led to serious injuries of even experienced backcountry travelers.
- When walking near the edges of bluffs or cliffs, watch for loose or crumbling rocks. Resist the temptation to go to the edge. Keep a safe distance from edges.
- Hurrying puts you at risk of falling. Slow down and enjoy the outing.
- Wear proper footwear, with soles to match the terrain.
- Use a bright light at night.

There are a lot more emergency calls made in the backcountry for fall victims each year than for snakebites, spider bites, and bear attacks combined. Use common sense as to where to climb or put your feet when on an outing.

BEAR ATTACK

One of the most common fears of inexperienced wilderness travelers is an attack from a bear. From time to time, people are indeed attacked by bears, both grizzly and black bears. In most cases, this is the fault of the people, not the bears, because bears don't normally hunt people. The most dangerous bears are those that have become accustomed to people, especially in parks,

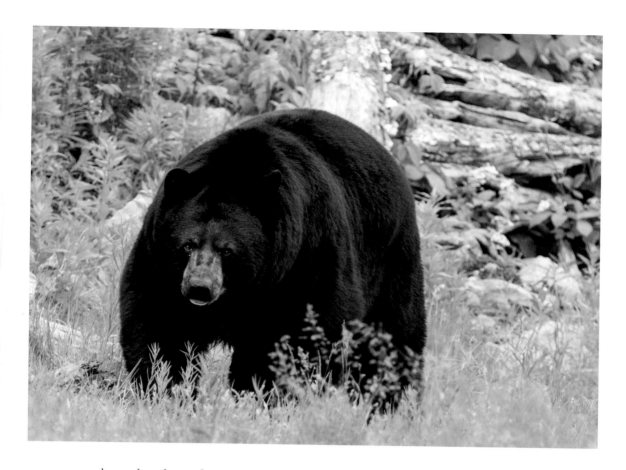

campgrounds, and garbage dumps. These bears have lost their fear of man and can be highly unpredictable.

Basically, bears like to keep their distance from humans, but when human and bear are suddenly thrown together, the result can be grim for the human. Anyone who accidentally gets between a grizzly sow and her cubs is in serious trouble, for example.

Bears shouldn't keep you from enjoying the outdoors, but when you are going into bear country, you should know what to do and what not to do in order to live in harmony with these powerful animals.

If planning a trip into bear country, obtain information about the area and if bears are found in the area. Much of the US is free of bears, so in these areas the bear threat is nonexistent. However, if bears are living in the area that you plan on traveling through, then a few precautions can keep you out of trouble.

Be Prepared for a Bear Encounter

If going into bear country, include a can of bear spray in your equipment and keep it where you can get to it quickly in the unlikely event it should be needed. Always select an EPA-approved product that is specifically designed to stop bears. Personal defense, jogger defense, law enforcement or military defense sprays may not contain the correct ingredients, or have the proper delivery system, to stop a charging bear.

Only use bear spray products that clearly state "for deterring attacks by bears." EPA-registered bear sprays have an active ingredient, clearly shown on the label, of 1 to 2 percent capsaicin and related capsaicinoids (found in chili peppers). This active ingredient is what affects the bear's eyes, nose, mouth, throat, and lungs.

EPA-registered bear sprays have a minimum duration of at least six seconds to compensate for multiple bears; wind; bears that may zigzag, circle, or charge multiple times; and for the hike out after you have stopped a charging bear.

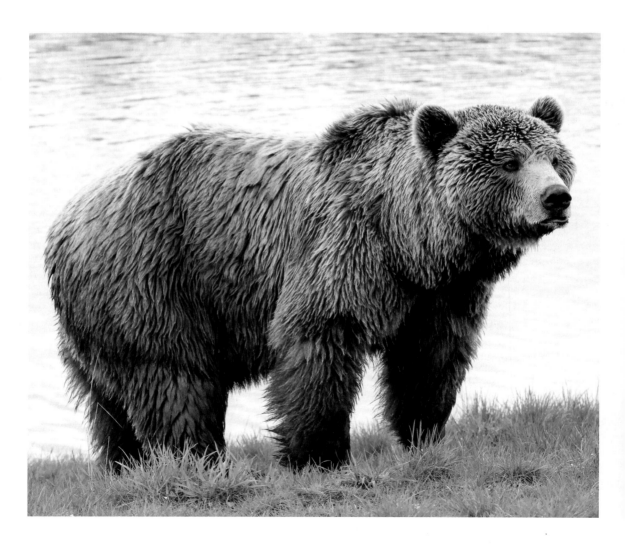

EPA-registered bear sprays shoot a minimum distance of twenty-five feet, a distance at which the active ingredients will reach the bear at sufficient strength to affect it in time to divert or stop the bear's charge and give it time to retreat.

Bear spray is intended to be sprayed into the face of an oncoming bear. Factors influencing effectiveness include distance, wind, rainy weather, temperature extremes, and product shelf life. It is not intended to act as a repellent. Do not spray gear or your camp with bear spray. Pre-sprayed objects may actually attract bears.

Visitors in bear country should carry a can of bear spray in an easily accessible fashion. Bear spray should also be readily available in the sleeping, cooking, and toilet areas of backcountry camps.

It's important to be sure the expiration date on your bear spray is current. It's equally important to study how to use it in advance and to follow the manufacturer's instructions. Know how to use the spray, and be aware of its limitations.

Leave the safety clip on the trigger unless you are ready to spray an aggressive bear. The spray may accidentally discharge otherwise. If you use the spray to stop a bear, leave the area immediately.

Under no circumstances should bear spray create a false sense of security or serve as a substitute for standard safety precautions in bear county.

If You Surprise a Bear in the Wild

Stand still, stay calm, and let the bear identify you and leave. Talk in a normal tone of voice. Be sure the bear has an escape route.

Never run or climb a tree.

If you see cubs, their mother is usually close by. Leave the area immediately.

If the Bear Doesn't Leave

A bear standing up is just trying to identify what you are by getting a better look and smell.

Wave your arms slowly overhead and talk calmly. If the bear huffs, pops its jaws, or stomps a paw, it wants you to give it space.

If on a trail, step off the trail to the downhill side, keep looking at the bear, and slowly back away until the bear is out of sight.

If the Bear Approaches

A bear knowingly approaching a person could be a food-conditioned bear looking for a handout or, very rarely, an aggressive bear. Stand your ground. Yell or throw small rocks in the direction of the bear. Don't feed him!

Get out your bear spray and use it when the bear is about forty feet away. Try to spray downwind, not upwind, so the spray doesn't blow back and get you.

If you're attacked, don't play dead. Fight back with anything available. People have successfully defended themselves with knives, hiking sticks, and even bare hands.

Keeping Bears Out of Camp

National Parks are likely to offer storage lockers or food poles at campsites; wilderness campsites will often require you to find your own tree suitable for hanging your food from. Bring at least thirty feet of rope or paracord and enough stuff sacks to hang your food, garbage, and scented items from food poles or trees. Plan on bringing at least one stuff sack for every two people in your group. Waterproof stuff sacks are best in case it rains. You can also seal everything inside your stuff sack into a smell-proof plastic bag to keep both the contents dry and the smells more contained.

Pick a tree that is at least one hundred yards from your survival camp. Hang your food sacks from a branch that is at least ten feet off the ground, with the sack hanging at least four feet from the trunk of the tree.

Bears will usually move out of the way if they hear people approaching, so make noise. Don't surprise bears! Bear bells are often not sufficient. Calling out (try saying "Hey Bear") and clapping your hands at regular intervals are better ways to make your presence known.

Some trail conditions make it hard for bears to hear, see, or smell approaching hikers. Be particularly careful near streams, when it's windy, in dense vegetation, or in any circumstance that limits line of sight (e.g. a blind corner or rise in the trail).

Never intentionally get close to a bear. Individual bears have their own personal space requirements that vary depending on their mood. Each bear will react differently, and a bear's behavior cannot be predicted. All bears are wild and dangerous and should be respected equally.

MOUNTAIN LION ATTACK

Mountain lions, sometimes called pumas or cougars, are making a comeback in many areas, but much of the US and Canada is free of mountain lions. As with bears, check to see if mountain lions are present in the area before you go on a backcountry outing. Even if they are, the chances of seeing one are very slim, and if you do, consider yourself special, as they are magnificent animals.

Should you encounter a mountain lion, here is what the Mountain Lion Foundation (www.mountainlion.org) recommends you should do:

- Stay back and take the encounter seriously.
- Seem as large as possible. Make yourself appear larger. Open your jacket, raise your arms slowly.
- Make noise, yell, shout, bang your walking stick or water bottle. Make any loud sound that cannot be confused by the lion as the sound of prey. Speak slowly and loudly to disrupt and discourage the lion's hunting instincts.
- Act defiant, not afraid. Maintain eye contact. Never run past or away from a mountain lion.
- Don't bend over or crouch down. Aggressively wave your arms, throw stones or branches, do not turn away.
- Slowly create distance. Assess the situation. Consider whether you may be between the lion and its kittens, prey, or cache. Back away slowly to give the mountain lion a path to retreat, never turning your back.
- Give the lion the time and ability to get away.

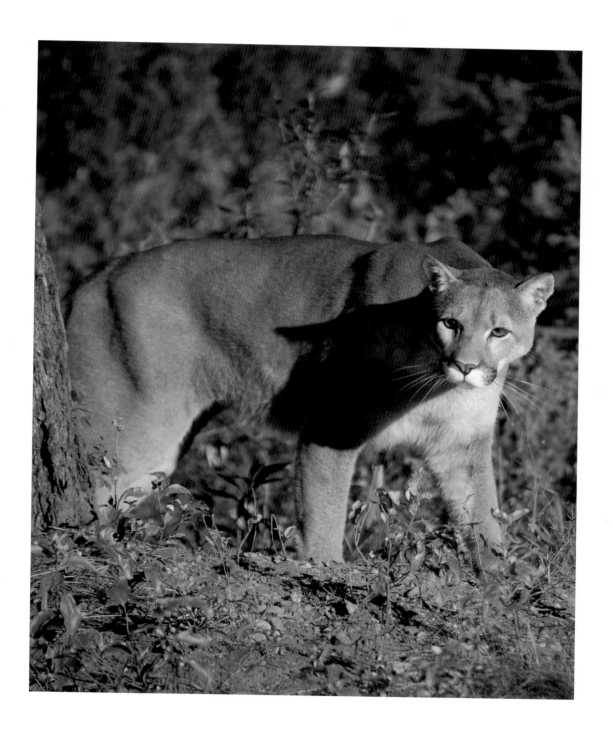

POTENTIAL DANGERS

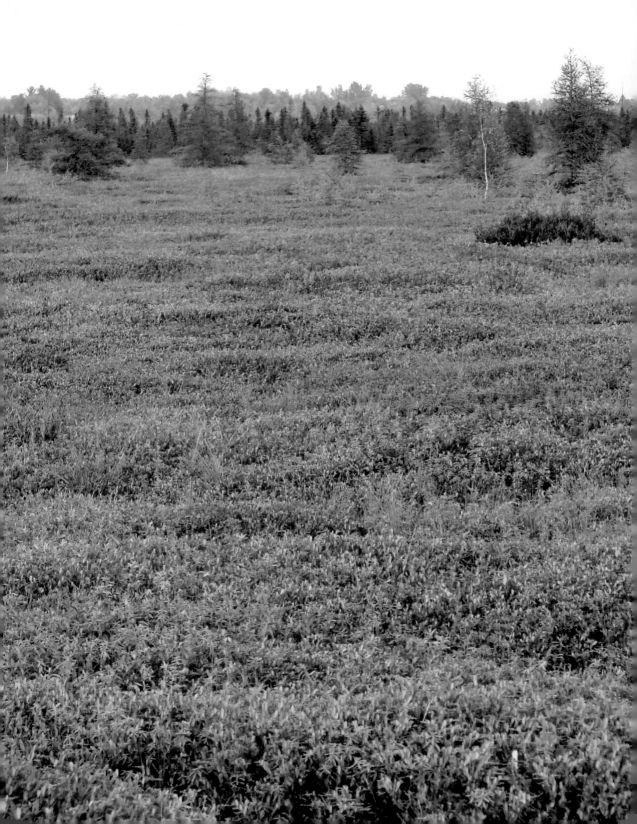

15

SURVIVE A VEHICLE STRANDING

Perhaps one of the most common strandings in North America is the broken-down automobile, truck, or SUV. We see them alongside our roads and highways every day. For the people involved, the stranding is usually nothing more a nuisance, as help is nearby. However, for those people who travel into little-traveled areas, such as national forest roads, and suddenly find themselves stranded, the situation can become serious quickly.

Anyone going anywhere with a vehicle—car, truck, ATV, trail bike, or snowmobile—should let someone know their plans. This is especially true if the trip, long or short, takes the vehicle off the beaten path. File a trip plan. Where are you going, when do you plan to arrive at your destination, when do you plan to return? If you should turn up missing, the authorities would have something to go on.

Always keep your vehicle in good working order by having it checked before trips. Fan belts account for many stranded situations each year, as does running out of fuel. Make sure your belts are in good shape and carry a spare with tools. Plan the fuel for your trips on the one-third tank rule: one-third tank going, one-third tank returning, and one-third tank in reserve.

If it is doubtful that your vehicle can make a trip, don't take it.

Watch the weather. Each winter we read of people who get caught in snow and ice storms and are found dead by rescue teams. Our need to go gets many of us in trouble every winter.

Listen to a weather report applicable for the area you will be traveling in before you depart on a trip. If the weather service reports storm warnings, stay home. If you get caught in a snow storm, stay with your vehicle. Have survival gear and rest up for rescue. If possible, keep the top of the vehicle free of snow so that it can be seen from the air. Carry a bright orange panel if your car color blends in with the snow.

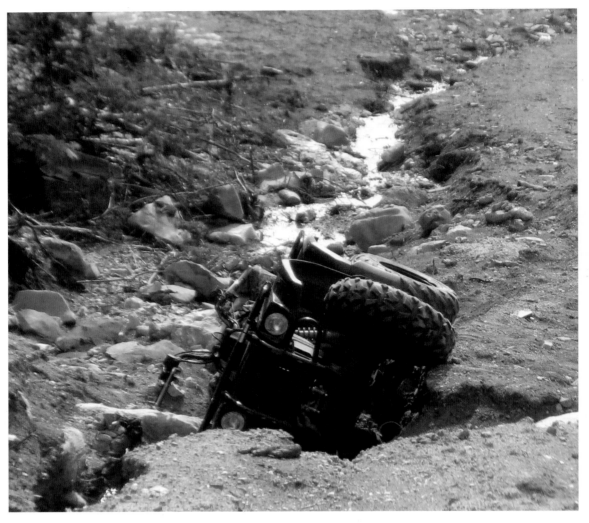

Even an ATV can get hopelessly stuck, resulting in the rider being stranded in a remote area.

CARRY SURVIVAL GEAR

Every vehicle should carry basic survival gear that is upgraded periodically to match the season and the terrain in which you will be traveling. A fully equipped survival kit should be carried. A well-charged cell phone should always be in any vehicle that doesn't have an on-board communications device.

Another vital survival item that all vehicles should carry is a portable air compressor. This handy device takes care of low tires on passenger vehicles, 4X4 vehicles, pickups, RVs, motorcycles, ATVs, and bicycles on the spot. It plugs into a vehicle's twelve-volt socket and usually has a long power cord and three-foot air hose. Some models are run on rechargeable batteries. There is a positive latching tire valve connector with pressure check stem to allow pressure checking without removing the connector from the tire. The air compressor fits compactly in the vehicle trunk or storage area.

Additional survival items that you should keep in your vehicle include a first aid kit, one gallon of water (much more if you are traveling in desert country), emergency food, matches in a waterproof container, basic tools for repairs, spare parts, tow rope, rain gear, shovel, ax, and, during cold weather, tire chains and one sleeping bag per person.

During cool or cold weather, your vehicle makes an excellent shelter and is easy to spot, so there is no need to leave it. Since most cars are tightly built, keep a window slightly open to allow oxygen to enter. This is especially true if you are burning anything in the car or running the motor to keep warm.

In extremely hot weather, the vehicle can become an oven. Seek shelter in the shade around or under the vehicle.

FOUR-WHEEL-DRIVE VEHICLES

My work in wildlife management brings me into contact each year with hundreds of sportsmen who are using four-wheel-drive vehicles to get into the backcountry. Many of these people are experienced outdoorsmen but are somewhat inexperienced in driving through mud, large rocks, and sand. I see scores of these vehicles stuck, and most could have avoided the problem.

A lot of new owners of four-wheelers, and there are thousands every year now, think just because they paid $60,000 for their vehicle and it has big tires, plus a winch, that it can swim through the deepest mud hole or fly over the largest rock pile. This attitude can only lead to trouble.

Let's start from the beginning and see how the driver of a four-wheel-drive vehicle should approach backcountry driving.

Get your vehicle ready for the trip. Proper tires should have round shoulders and a moderately aggressive tread such as the standard mud-grip or all-weather tread. You should have a power winch installed if your budget can stand the cost. You should also have a tool chest that includes snow chains (even though you don't expect snow), shovel, ax, compact air compressor, two jacks, fifty-foot nylon rope for towing (10,000-pound test), two two-inch-thick by one-foot-wide by two-foot-long planks, and a set of wrenches.

If you don't have a winch, be sure and add what's known as a "come-along" to your tool chest. The come-along is simply a hand-powered winch. It is best described as a hand-cranked, cable-filled wheel and ratchet. You attach one end of the cable to a tree and the come-along to the vehicle frame. Each time you pump the handle, the wheel takes up the cable, winching you out of the mud hole.

Once you leave maintained roads, the trick is to travel slowly and study the road carefully. If there is any doubt about the condition of the road ahead, stop, get out of your vehicle, and do a little walking. How deep is the mud, or how deep is the hole under the water? Use a stick and test each situation. Common sense should tell you when to turn around and find a new route.

If the going looks as though it's going to get rough, put on your tire chains. They work as well in slick mud as they do in snow. Another trick to use, especially in deep sand, is to decrease your tire pressure to approximately twelve pounds. This allows your tires to "float." Don't forget to inflate them again as you get out of the trouble area.

Learn to use your winch (or your come-along) before you actually need it. Numerous times I have come upon a shiny new four-wheel-drive vehicle stuck and found that the owner did not know how to use his winch. When you buy your winch, make sure the salesman gives you a good session in its proper and safe use.

The most frustrating situation, and one of the most common emergencies that four-wheelers find themselves in, is to have all four wheels stuck, unable to move forward or backward. If you have an electric winch, the solution is to hook the cable to a tree and throw the switch. If you don't have a winch, then hook up your come-along and be prepared to sweat a little. Use your shovel to clear the way for each tire to move. If you don't have either of these devices, a third possibility is to get an accompanying vehicle to pull you out.

If you have none of these options, you are in for some work. You must shovel away all the mud that's piled up underneath the vehicle. This is supporting the weight of the chassis and keeping weight off the tires, thereby causing the tires to lose traction.

Once you have the vehicle's under-carriage free of mud, get out a jack and plank. Using the plank as a platform for the jack, raise the wheel that is deepest in the mud. Dig out the mud beneath the wheel down to a firm base. Then fill up the hole with rocks, logs, brush, and such. Now lower the wheel slowly down onto the firm platform you've constructed. Do the same thing to each of the other wheels. Then extend the solid platforms for several feet in front of each wheel. If you don't, you'll be able to move forward only a few feet and then will be back into the same predicament.

Sandy areas should be traveled over with caution. The important thing to remember in sand or soft dirt is to keep moving steadily and not too fast. Don't apply an excess of power that would cause the wheels to dig in. Try to avoid abrupt changes in speed or direction, and aim as straight as possible across the area. Avoid sharp turns, as sharp turns cause the front tires to scrub sideways, turning them into plows that can raise impassable pileups of the sand. It would take a book to list the various ways people get stuck in the backcountry with their vehicles and the ways to get them out. If only they would learn the capabilities and limits of their vehicles and how to read backcountry roads, most of these situations would be avoided. Unavoidable pitfalls can be remedied in a short time by knowing how to use your emergency equipment and applying it with a little common sense.

THE VEHICLE AS A SURVIVAL TOOL

The vehicle can aid your survival in many ways. The mirrors can be used for signaling. The battery can produce sparks for fire starting. The cigarette lighter can start proper burning for fire starting. Hubcaps can be used for shovels or buckets or cooking vessels. Floor mats can be used to give wheels traction to get unstuck. The spare tire can be used as a seat to get you up off hot sand or burned for a smoke signal. Wiring from a car can be used for snares. The list could go on and on.

The vehicle can provide you with a vast variety of survival tools, but if you carry the proper survival gear this will not have to be necessary.

IF A BLIZZARD TRAPS YOU IN YOUR CAR

If you get caught in a snow storm, stay with your vehicle. Have survival gear and rest up for rescue. If possible, keep the top of the vehicle free of snow so that it can be seen from the air. Carry a bright orange panel if your car color blends in with the snow. Here are some rules to follow:

- Stay in the vehicle. Do not attempt to walk in a blizzard. Disorientation comes quickly in blowing and drifting snow. Being lost in open country during a blizzard is extremely dangerous. You are more likely to be found in your car and will at least be sheltered there.
- Avoid overexertion and exposure. Exertions from attempting to push your car, shoveling heavy drifts, and performing other difficult chores during strong winds, blinding snow, and bitter cold of a blizzard may cause a heart attack—even for persons in apparently good physical condition.
- Keep a downwind window slightly open for fresh air. Freezing rain, wet snow, and wind-driven snow can completely seal the passenger compartment.
- Beware of carbon monoxide. Run the engine, heater, or catalytic heater sparingly, and only with a downwind window open for ventilation. Make sure that snow has not blocked the exhaust pipe.
- Exercise by clapping your hands and moving your arms and legs vigorously from time to time, and do not stay in one position for long. But don't overdo it. Exercise warms you, but it also increases body heat loss.
- If more than one person is in the vehicle, don't sleep at the same time. Take turns keeping watch for searchers.
- Turn on the dome light occasionally at night to make sure your vehicle is more visible to working or search crews.
- Don't panic. Stay with the car.

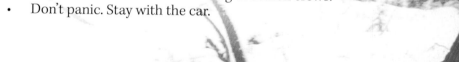

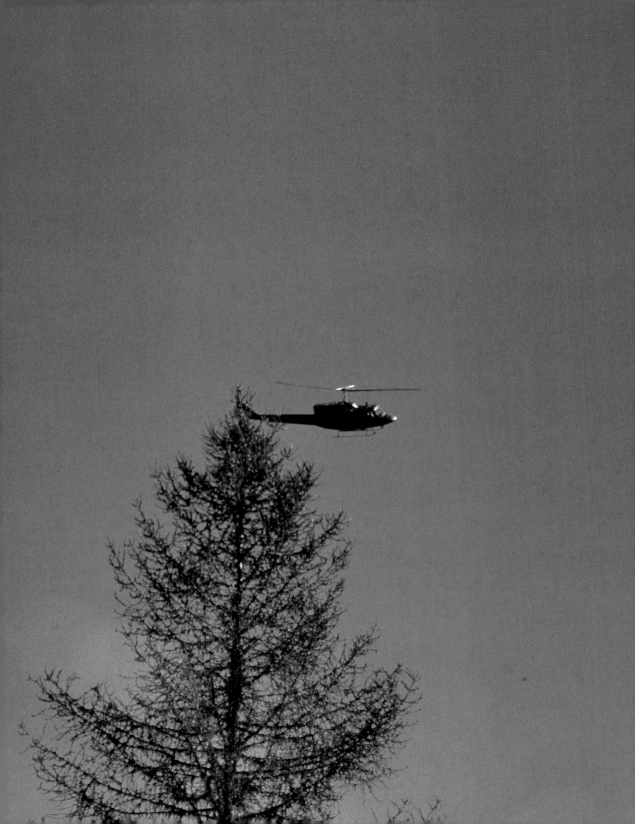

16

DOWNED AIRCRAFT SURVIVAL

"Mayday, Mayday, Mayday." This emergency code comes in from many airplanes in trouble. In fact, the Civil Air Patrol participates an average of one thousand search missions each year, most of which are for downed aircraft. Most of the people in these aircraft never thought it would happen to them. One minute they were comfortably flying over rough, remote terrain, the next minute they were on the ground in a survival situation.

According to the Civil Air Patrol, of every one hundred persons involved in air crashes, only thirty-five will survive initially, only eighteen will survive for twenty-four hours, and fewer than ten will live more than seventy-two hours.

Some of the after-crash deaths can be avoided. With the proper survival gear, survival training, and a will to live, many of these people could live for days or weeks.

WHAT TO DO BEFORE YOU FLY
Before anyone, either passenger or pilot, takes off on a private plane trip, he should make sure that a few basic rules are followed.

File a flight plan
Be sure a flight plan is filed, and stay with the plan. If you change your plans while flying, notify the Federal Aviation Administration (FAA) of this change at once. Upon arrival at your destination, file an arrival report. Remember that a search normally starts after you fail to report in and enough time has passed that your fuel is exhausted—usually about three hours. Don't delay the arrival report.

When no flight plan is filed, the rescue attempt can be delayed for a long time or may never happen.

Check the Emergency Locator Transmitter
The Emergency Locator Transmitter (ELT), usually located in the tail of the aircraft, has proven to be the best aid to searchers and the best hope for timely rescue of survivors of air crashes.

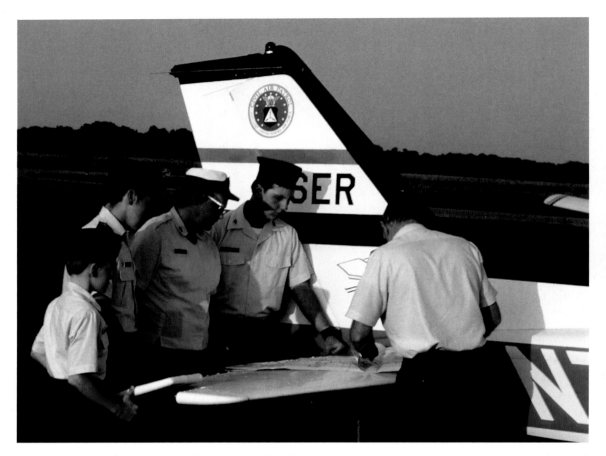

Once an aircraft is reported missing, the Civil Air Patrol jumps into action and a logical search is begun immediately.

The ELT is a small electronic box which can beam out a strong signal when activated. It is activated upon the plane's impact with the ground. This signal can be picked up by commercial and military aircraft. It can also be picked up by satellites that are carrying a SARSAT (Search and Rescue Satellite Aided Tracking) package. With the aid of the SARSAT satellites, the science of finding aircraft and oceangoing vessels in distress has taken a giant step. Don't fly in a plane that doesn't have an ELT.

Carry Survival Gear

Be sure your plane has a survival kit and survival gear. The survival gear should be stored in a daypack so that it will be kept together in the plane, making it easy to retrieve after a crash and easy to carry if you must change locations. Don't forget to include food and water in your survival gear. You could be in for a long wait.

Dress and Equip Yourself According to Ground Weather

It is important for you to dress according to the ground weather you will be flying over. You may choose to dress in light clothing because you may be going from warm airport to warm plane to warm airport. However, if you're forced down in cold mountains along the way, you don't have much of a chance of survival. If you don't want to wear the clothing, at least take it with you. A sleeping bag per person should be taken during cold weather. Rain gear should be taken during wet weather.

Watch the weather along the entire route and cancel or postpone the trip if there is any question concerning the weather or changes in weather. If your route takes you over large bodies of water, take along a self-inflatable life raft and know how to use it.

When You Go Down

Here are steps to take if your aircraft goes down:

1. Get the survival gear and exit the aircraft immediately (thus the reason to have it packed in a day pack).
2. Move everyone a safe distance from the aircraft to avoid dangers from fire and explosions. Wait until the engines have cooled and spilled aviation fuel has evaporated before returning to the aircraft.
3. Treat the injured as quickly as possible.
4. While awaiting your return to the aircraft, make temporary shelter to protect everyone from inclement weather.
5. Get signals ready for use in the event searchers reach the area quickly.
6. Reassure everyone, including yourself, and remain calm.
7. If the aircraft radios are still serviceable, they should momentarily be tuned to the distress frequency to ensure that the ELT is operating. Once the ELT is activated, it must be left on, since turning it off can result in a search aircraft being thwarted in its attempt to home in on the transmission.
8. If the aircraft radios are operational, try to make contact with the FAA on a local frequency.
9. Search the aircraft for items that you may have to use in survival—maps, clothing, tools.
10. At this point, a major decision must be reached, and that is whether to stay with the aircraft or leave the crash site. The basic rule is to stay with the aircraft if at all possible, since searchers will be looking for it soon and because it has an ELT working for you. You will also avoid the possible hazards of travel. Your chances will be good if you have made radio contact; if you have come down on course or near a traveled air route; or if weather and air observation conditions are good.
11. The aircraft is generally easier to spot from the air than by people traveling on foot. Someone may even have seen your plane go down and may be along to investigate. The aircraft or parts from it can provide you with shelter, signaling aids, and other equipment. If the temperature is neither too cold nor too hot, the cabin of the plane can be used a shelter. However, in temperature extremes, the cabin can be an oven or refrigerator. If

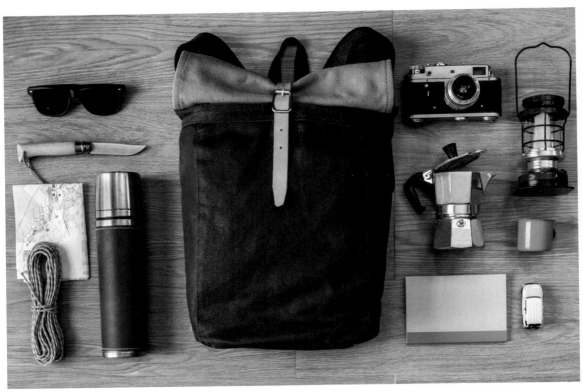

If your aircraft is downed, gather anything that you think you may need for survival purposes.

the weather is cold, the plane's insulation and upholstery can be used to make items such as sleeping bags, caps, or mattresses. Wings, rudders, or doors may be used to make shelter. The battery can provide a spark for fire-starting. Such items as maps, curtains, and newspapers can be used to improve the shelter and to provide warmth. Use cowling for reflector signals, tubing for shelter framework, and the generator for radio power.

There are rare occasions, however, when you may need to move some distance from the aircraft, such as if it is down under trees and cannot be seen from the air, as in the classic case of Helen Klaben and Ralph Flores. The pair left Whitehorse, Yukon, heading for San Francisco in a small private airplane, neither had survival training. Over the Yukon-British Columbia border, they ran into a blinding snowstorm which caused them to crash.

For over a month, search and rescue aircraft flew over the area looking for the downed plane, but the thick trees in which Helen and Ralph had crashed hid the plane from view.

Both Helen and Ralph were injured in the crash, but they managed to set up a survival camp at the aircraft. They had very little survival gear on the plane: matches, a little food, some vitamin pills, two tubes of toothpaste, a hammer, cold chisel, hunting knife, books, canvas motor cover,

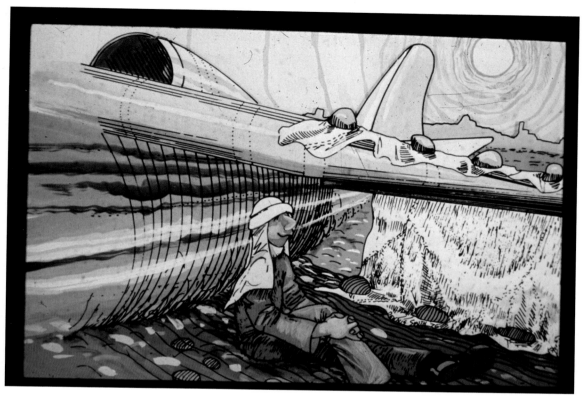

Stay with the downed aircraft if it is safe to do so, as this is where the searchers will be looking.

and extra clothing. For a blanket, they tore the carpet from the plane floor and insulation from the walls and ceiling. Seat and back cushions were used for beds. Firewood was cut with the chisel and hammer. During their ordeal, temperatures dropped to -40 F.

Their food ran out the first week. From then on, it was only water, which they got by melting snow in a can. Their drinking cup was made from a light reflector from the plane. They made several attempts to kill rabbits that came near their camp, but nothing worked.

For thirty-three days they stayed with the aircraft, but after hearing forty to fifty aircraft pass nearby, they decided they must move if they were to be found. On snowshoes made from branches and a toboggan made from aircraft parts, they moved their meager supplies through deep snow to an opening in the forest. Since they were very weak, this three-quarters-of-a-mile journey was quite tough. Here they used the engine cover tarpaulin to make a tent. Ralph then moved to another clearing about two miles distant and tramped SOS in the snow, as well as an arrow aimed in Helen's direction. Also, they placed in the snow a fragment of their plane which showed the plane's identification number.

This new camp and signals resulted in their being found. A bush pilot flying supplies to trappers spotted the SOS and the arrow, and then Helen and Ralph. They were rescued forty-nine days after crashing into the frozen wilderness.

If your aircraft is hidden, the first thing to do is try to cut trees and brush to make it visible from the air. If this is impossible, move only a short distance to the first clearing you can find, and set up your ground-to-air sign.

Organize for Rescue

If you are with a group of survivors, organize them and your camp so that everyone who is able will stay busy and the camp will be prepared for comfort until rescue arrives.

The first step in organizing is to appoint individual members to specific jobs, based on their abilities and their physical and mental capacities to handle them. With one person in charge, pool all food and equipment. Prepare a shelter to protect everyone from rain, sand, snow, wind, cold, or insects. Collect all possible firewood, the variety of which will be determined by your geographical location. Always try to have at least one day's supply of wood on hand. Then look for water. Make sure your signals are always in good shape and ready for instant use.

Reassure everyone, and try to keep the will to live alive even if rescue is several days in coming. As we saw in the beginning of this chapter, many survivors of aircraft crashes die while waiting for rescue. This is an unnecessary loss of life. By carrying the necessary survival gear, taking precautions such as filing flight plans, learning survival techniques, and using survival skills when the aircraft is down, you should make it through aircraft survival situations.

At no time attempt to move unless you know exactly where you are and where you are going. To wander aimlessly uses up vital energy that is very difficult to replace under survival conditions. If you are leaving a crash site, even for a short distance, leave a message for rescuers indicating the date and direction of your travel. Regardless of your reason for moving, consider the weather. Stay put if adverse weather would further endanger you. If travel for help is indicated, send the most fit people—two, if possible. To travel alone is dangerous.

Make a definite plan to follow. Determine the nearest rescue point, the distance to it, the possible difficulties and hazards of travel, and the facilities and supplies at the destination. Travel is extremely risky unless you have the necessities of survival to support you during travel. You should have sufficient water to reach the next possible source of water as indicated on your map or chart, enough food to last until you are able to procure additional food, and a means of shelter.

While this chapter has given some pointers on traveling away from the crash site, such travel is not usually recommended. The most important rule of downed aircraft survival is to stay with the aircraft.

17

SURVIVING VARIOUS ENVIRONMENTS

Hiking, backpacking, wilderness exploring, conservation projects, fishing, hunting, canoeing, and a vast number of other outings can carry a person into environments that are different than what they are accustomed to or are totally foreign to them. Each of these environments has its own weather patterns, terrain, vegetated cover, and challenges. Survival in each of these environments increases with the knowledge of the environment and how well the outing is planned using this knowledge.

WOODLANDS

Across North America there are a wide variety of woodlands ranging from wet rainforest to semi-arid brush country. Most people think of woodlands as park-like places containing a wealth of survival materials for making shelter, fire, signals, and finding water. While in some cases that is true, that may not be the case in others or in severe weather conditions. A rainstorm can make everything wet and difficult to use. Some rainforests are that way most of the time.

Heavy woodlands can have a thick canopy, making signaling to aircraft almost impossible and their seeing you very difficult. Finding an opening may be difficult or you may have to create one. A heavily canopied woodland is one place a signal fire is most valuable, as thick smoke may find its way to the top of the canopy, where searchers can see it. Care must be taken with the fire, as you don't want to start a forest fire. You have enough problems without that.

Damp woodlands can be cold even in the deep South. Some woodlands get heavy snow, which can make travel almost impossible and survival become a race to stay warm and dry.

In a semi-arid forest, finding water can be near impossible, while forest where there is plenty of water may be swarming with mosquitoes or blackflies by the millions, depending on the season. Be prepared.

In flat woodlands, keeping a sense of direction can be nearly impossible without navigational aids. On a cloudy day, woodlands of this type are the easiest to get lost in, even near home.

Here are some tips to consider when planning a trip into woodlands:

- Study the woodlands you plan on going into. Get to know the woods for the season and weather when you plan your outing.
- Study topo maps of the woods and plan your trip carefully. Take the map, compass, and GPS with you.
- File a trip plan.
- Get a weather forecast for the period you plan on being in the woods.
- Dress for the weather and the conditions you anticipate. Carry clothing for unexpected weather such as rain or a drop in temperature. Wear correct boots for the conditions.
- Carry insect repellent in your survival kit, plus extra repellent if the area is known for mosquitoes or blackflies.
- Use navigational aids from the very beginning of the trip. To get lost in a vast, flat hardwood bottom is the wrong time to break out the map and compass.

MOUNTAINS

The mountain environment, whether it is in the southern Appalachians of Georgia or the Brooks Range of Alaska, can be one of sudden weather changes. In the Cassiar Mountains of British Columbia, within one hour I have seen warm sunshine, rain, sleet, and heavy snow. In the Snowbird Mountains of North Carolina, I have seen weather go from a bright, bluebird day to a fierce electrical storm with little advance warning.

Mountain Dangers

The basic rule of mountain survival is to understand the dangers of the mountains, put a lot of planning into any trip into the mountains, and go prepared. If a survival crisis should occur in the mountains, travel should be halted as soon as is practical. Rarely can you improve your lot by trying to struggle out of the mountains. It is usually wiser to establish a position where you can be easily seen and then await rescue.

Falls

Falls and the survival situations resulting from falls probably account for more search and rescue efforts in the mountain environment than any other hazard. These mishaps can occur not only to those involved in the seemingly more dangerous mountain sports, such as mountain climbing, rappelling, and other rock-climbing activities, but to anyone exploring, hiking, fishing, or hunting in a mountainous terrain. Even a relaxing afternoon of fly fishing in a beautiful mountain stream can become deadly if a sudden fall breaks a hip.

A fall in the mountains is a life-threatening occurrence. You cannot be too careful to avoid this very real and ever-present danger.

Lightning

The fiercest electrical storm I have ever witnessed occurred the first year that I guided in Colorado. I had a pack string of animals above timberline one afternoon when, without warning, an electrical storm hit. Lightning was popping the rocks along the mountaintop on which we were riding. The horses were going crazy, and there was little for us riders to do but get off, go down the side of the mountain, spread out, and lie flat on the ground. The storm lasted for almost an hour. It was one of the most frightening hours I have ever spent.

Electrical storms are to be expected in mountains during the warm months, accompanied by large hail. You must keep a constant eye on the weather and make an effort to drop below timberline or get out from under high trees when an electrical storm is approaching. Although thunderstorms are local in nature and usually short in duration, they can be a real threat.

Wind

In high mountains, the ridges and passes are seldom calm. But in protected alleys, strong winds are rare. Normally, wind velocity increases with altitude, since the earth's frictional drag is strongest near the ground, and this effect is accentuated by mountainous terrain. Winds are accelerated when they are forced over ridges and peaks or when they converge through mountain passes and canyons. Because of these funneling effects, the winds may blast with greater force on an exposed mountainside or summit. In most cases, the local wind direction is controlled by topography.

The force exerted by wind quadruples each time the wind speed doubles; that is, wind blowing at 40 miles per hour pushes four times harder than does wind blowing 20 miles per hour. At increasing wind strengths, gusts become more important and may be 50 percent higher than average wind velocity. Always have a place to seek shelter if the wind speed increases.

Dehydration

High mountain air is dry, especially in winter when the humidity in the air condenses into ice. This dryness increases with the altitude. The amount of vapor in the air decreases in geometric proportion as the altitude increases. Consequently, dehydration is a common problem with people in the mountains. Drink water, even if you aren't thirsty, to avoid this condition.

Flash Floods

Since many mountains receive heavy rainfall, particularly near the top, flash flooding is common. It is not unusual for a pleasant brook to suddenly become a rushing wall of water. When camping, keep flash floods in mind. Especially when you are under the stress of a survival situation, avoid setting up your camp close to a creek, low drainage depression, or in a dry wash, as you may be placing yourself in the path of a flash flood.

Snow

Snow can cause many problems for winter mountain travelers, including hampered travel. Many times each fall, news reports from Rocky Mountain states announce that hunters are snowed in and that rescue efforts are under way.

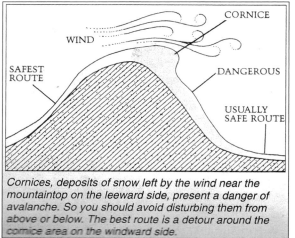

Cornices, deposits of snow left by the wind near the mountaintop on the leeward side, present a danger of avalanche. So you should avoid disturbing them from above or below. The best route is a detour around the cornice area on the windward side.

Associated with snow slopes is the avalanche. Even small avalanches can have tremendous force and are a serious threat. Snow avalanches are complex natural phenomena. Since experts do not fully understand all the causes, it is difficult to predict avalanche conditions with certainty.

The more time you spend in high country skiing, snowshoeing, snowmobiling, and engaged in other winter activities, the greater are your chances of being caught by an avalanche.

Survival in Avalanche Areas

The safest routes are on ridgetops and slightly on the windward side away from cornices. Windward slopes are usually safer than leeward slopes. If you cannot travel on ridges, the next safest route is out in the valley, far from the bottom of slopes subject to descent of avalanches.

Avoid disturbing cornices from below or above. Gain ridgetops by detouring around cornice areas.

If you must cross dangerous slopes, stay high and near the top. If you see avalanche fracture lines in the snow, avoid them and similar snow areas.

If you must ascend or descend a dangerous slope, go straight up or down; do not make traverses back and forth across the slope.

Take advantage of areas of dense timber, ridges, or rocky outcrops as islands of safety. Use them for lunch and rest stops. Spend as little time as possible on open slopes.

Snowmobiles should not cross the lower part of the slopes. Do not drive a snowmobile across especially long, open slopes or known avalanche paths.

Obey posted signs put up by authorities, closing slopes because of danger. If you must cross a dangerous slope, only one person at a time should cross. All others should watch. To cross a dangerous slope, remove ski pole straps and ski safety straps, loosen all equipment, put on mitts and cap, and fasten clothing before you travel.

Authorities now recommend that all members of a party in avalanche country carry transceivers, which are pocket-size devices that can transmit and receive signals. When crossing avalanche-prone terrain, all members of the party switch into the transmit mode. Then, if one or more members are caught and buried, other members switch into the receive mode and home in on the victims. Probe poles that can be assembled in sections are also highly useful in probing for victims.

If you are caught in an avalanche:

- Discard all equipment.
- Get away from your snowmobile.

- Make swimming motions. Try to stay on top; work your way to the side of the avalanche.
- Before coming to a stop, get your hands in front of your face and try to make an air space in the snow.
- Try to remain calm.

If you are the survivor:

- Mark the place where you last saw victims.
- Search for victims directly downslope below the last seen point; if they are not on the surface, probe the snow with a pole or stick.
- Do not desert victims and go for help, unless help is only a few minutes away.

Remember, you must consider not only the time required for you to get help, but the time required for help to return. After thirty minutes, the buried victim has only a 50 percent chance of surviving.

If there is more than one survivor:

- Send one for help while the others search for the victim.
- Have the one who goes for help switch his transceiver to transmit mode, in case he gets buried by another avalanche. He should also mark the route effectively so a rescue party can follow back.
- Contact the ski patrol, local sheriff, or Forest Service.
- Administer first aid.
- Treat for suffocation and shock.

For information on the existence of possible avalanche conditions in an area, check the local weather forecasts and contact the Forest Service snow ranger or the nearest winter sports area ski patrol.

Mountain Trip Planning

Anytime you are going into the mountains, the trip should be planned carefully. The route taken, the condition of the roads to and from the mountains, the short-range and long-range weather forecast, and all other aspects of the trip should be carefully researched.

If it is an outing in bear country, check ahead to see if there are any bear warnings or trail closures due to bear problems.

Allow plenty of time for your trip. Often people think that they can accomplish many goals in the mountains in a day or two and return, not realizing that the steepness of the terrain, the elevation, and sudden changes in weather can all cause the trip to take much longer than expected.

Remember to set your limit and to know when to turn back when any member of the group cannot safely continue. The mountain will still be there for another day.

The majority of people I have guided on high mountain outings have not been in shape for the rigors of the trip. Also, you must be acclimated to the higher elevation. Coming from a city located near sea level and trying to climb a mountain that is over 10,000 feet high within a day or two is almost impossible and downright dangerous. In addition, fatigue causes bad judgment and carelessness, both of which have killed many people in the mountains.

In planning your trip, be sure that you have the proper equipment for the terrain and for the weather conditions that you can expect. Early in my career, I learned a hard lesson about wearing the right equipment in the Rocky Mountains. For quite some time I resisted buying a cowboy hat. I didn't want to look like a character from a Zane Grey novel on the high mountain trails. The local guides I was working with kept telling me that the day would come when I would wish I had a cowboy hat. I realized just how right they were one afternoon when a violent hailstorm hit our packstring. There was nowhere to go, and my head, face, and neck took a tremendous beating as golf ball-sized hail pounded us for fifteen minutes. Needless to say, as soon as I arrived back in civilization, I bought a cowboy hat.

Choose all mountain equipment carefully. If you doubt your ability to select the right equipment, get advice from someone who knows the area you are going into and who is an outfitter.

DESERTS

Travel in hot, dry deserts can be an enjoyable outing to those who are adequately prepared and knowledgeable as to its possible hazards. To the unprepared, though, it can be a horrible experience.

Walking

When in the desert, even travelers in good physical condition should walk slowly and rest about ten minutes per hour. At this rate, a person in good physical condition can initially cover about ten to twelve miles per day. After he becomes fatigued or if he lacks sufficient water or food, this distance becomes less.

Walking at night may be a good idea, because it is cooler then, and if lack of water is a problem, you will dehydrate less. However, the disadvantages are that you may not be able to see the ground well enough and may stumble or overlook water or food sources or signs of habitation. Another factor to consider in the desert is that rattlesnakes are active at night, so you may get too close to one without even realizing it, until you hear the telltale rattle. It is usually best to travel in the desert in early morning or late evening, spending midday in whatever shade may be available. Also, the position of the sun early and late in the day will give you a better sense of direction.

Pick the easiest and safest way to walk. Go around obstacles instead of over them. Rather than going up or down steep slopes, zigzag to prevent undue exertion. Go around gullies and canyons instead of through them. Watch for snakes, especially at night, because the desert is home to many rattlesnakes. When walking in sand, lean well forward, keeping your knees bent. When walking with companions, adjust the rate to the slowest person.

During breaks, try to sit down in the shade and prop your feet up high, remove your shoes and change socks, or straighten the ones you are wearing. If the ground is too hot to sit on, no shade is available, and you cannot raise your feet, do not remove your shoes, because you may not be able to get them back onto swollen feet. However, you can unlace boots or shoes, adjust socks, and re-lace.

Since shade may not be easy to find in a desert environment, the desert survival kit should contain a metallic plastic sheet, such as the MCR Medical Emergency Blanket. This silver sheet folds up to the size of a deck of playing cards and can be unfolded into a quick shade shelter by attaching it to rocks or brush with cord. Due to its silver color, it also serves as a signal, and at night, when the temperature drops, you can wrap up in it to stay warm.

Driving

Driving can be hazardous on little-used desert roads, but if a few simple suggestions are followed, desert driving can be done safely. Have a map of the area you are going into. Obtain current information from the highway patrol, conservation officer, or county sheriff's office as to the conditions of the roads in that area. Have a vehicle that is in good condition that is designed for off-road travel. Drive slowly. If in doubt about the terrain, stop and check it out first on foot. Do not attempt to drive on questionable roads without first checking the footing and clearances. High centers on rocks may rupture the oil pan. Washes may cause the powered wheels to become suspended above the ground.

In sand, the wheels may sink, resulting in a high center and loss of traction. Avoid spinning wheels to gain motion, because this will only cause the wheels to dig in further. Instead, apply power very slowly. Consider reducing tire pressure before you get in too deep.

Under emergency conditions, when driving in sand, traction can be increased by partially deflating tires. Be careful not to remove so much air that the tire may slip on the rim. Then, drive slowly. Start, stop, and turn gradually because sudden motions cause wheels to dig in.

Be sure to take these tools and equipment if you intend to drive off the main roads: one or more shovels, a pick, a tow chain or cable, at least fifty feet of strong nylon tow rope, portable air compressor, ax, full water containers, at least two full gas cans, extra fan belts, and your regular spare parts and auto tools. Include a survival kit and a tarp or means of creating a large area of shade. Be sure that your fuel tank is full, and that you have a filled, clean radiator, a filled battery, and new fan belts. If you become stuck or your car breaks down, raise the hood and stay with the car. The raised hood is an indication to other desert travelers that you need help.

Your vehicle can provide you with life-saving shade. In fact, one of the best shelters you can utilize if you are stranded is your vehicle. First of all, don't get into the vehicle because it will be like an oven. What you want is a double layer of insulation between the sun and you, and your car or truck can provide this. Here's how to construct a shelter:

1. Open all of the vehicle doors and windows for ventilation. Disconnect interior car lights that come on when doors are open. This will conserve the battery for other uses.
2. Using a shovel, board, or hubcap, scoop the dirt out from under the vehicle, away from the motor, tailpipe, or muffler, as they will all be hot. Dig away the top fifteen inches or more, the deeper the cooler.
3. Be sure to dig under the side or end of the vehicle where the shade is.
4. Take your time and avoid getting too hot.
5. Once you have the trench dug, crawl in and enjoy the shade. The ground temperature down fifteen inches deep should not be more than the mid-80s.

6. Be sure you have your ground-to-air signals out, and stay alert for rescue aircraft. If you decide to work on your vehicle or enlarge your shelter, wait until the cool of the evening.

Since the roof of the vehicle takes much of the sun's heat and the floor of the vehicle takes the secondary heat, the space under the vehicle can be one of the best shelters in the desert. Stay with your vehicle. Desert search and rescue experts state that many desert deaths occur within two hours after the victim leaves his shelter.

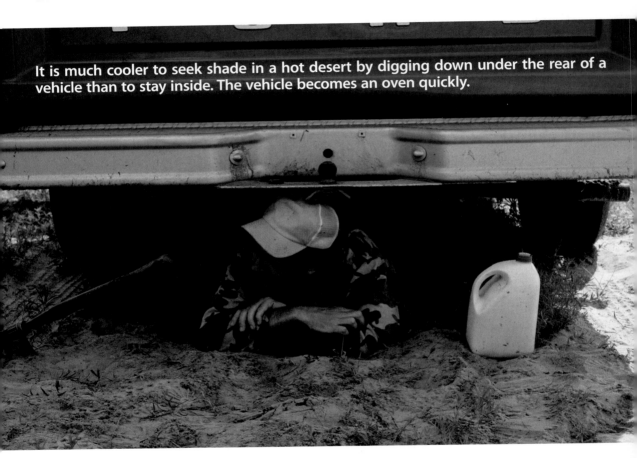

It is much cooler to seek shade in a hot desert by digging down under the rear of a vehicle than to stay inside. The vehicle becomes an oven quickly.

Dress for the Environment

In the desert, you should wear light-colored clothing to reflect some of the heat of the sun. Be sure to keep your clothing on, as clothing helps ration your sweat by slowing the evaporation rate and prolonging the cooling effect. It also helps keep out the hot desert air. Long-sleeve shirts and broad-brimmed hats are also recommended

Remember that deserts can be cold during the night, so a jacket in your daypack could be a welcome item of clothing if an unplanned night in the desert occurs.

Basic Rules for Desert Survival

By following a few basic rules, you can assure yourself of a safer trip into the desert:

1. Never go into the desert without filing a trip plan with responsible adults. Stick to the plan.
2. Carry at least one gallon of water per person per day.
3. Watch the weather. Even though a desert is a dry environment, flash floods can occur rapidly even if the rain may not fall where you are. Avoid travel in low areas if thunderstorms are on the horizon.
4. Carry a survival kit and a means of constructing quick shade.
5. Stay hydrated.
6. If water is limited, keep your mouth shut and breathe through your nose. Keep talking to a minimum, do not eat, and do not take salt.
7. Do not sit or lie directly on the ground, which may be 30 F degrees hotter than the air. Sit on your daypack.
8. A roadway is a sign of civilization. If you find a road, stay on it, for there's a good chance that help will happen along.
9. Always carry a charged cell phone.
10. If you become lost or stranded, stay put in the shade and put out signals.

RIVERS, LAKES, OCEAN

The ability to survive on streams and large bodies of water varies greatly, from a kayak trip on a creek to an offshore fishing trip on a large boat. The one thing they all have in common is in the planning.

Open bodies of water, be they rivers, lakes, or oceans, are subject to become dangerous quickly due to changes in the weather, such as thunderstorms bringing lightning, wind, and heavy rain, all which can make travel dangerous. Because of this, always check out the weather forecasts for the dates of your float trip or offshore excursion. During the trip, a sharp eye should always be kept on the weather.

Wear and carry clothing that is appropriate for the weather and wet conditions you may encounter. Hypothermia is a real threat for trips on water. In Nunavut Territory Canada not long ago, I got severe hypothermia just from the spray of a motorboat on a huge lake.

Regardless of whether a float trip is a half-day trip down a local river or an overnight deep-sea fishing excursion, a trip plan needs to be filed with responsible people.

For canoe, kayak, raft, and rowboat trips that require paddling or rowing, every member of the group should be in decent physical condition for the trip. These types of trips demand that you use muscles that you probably don't use otherwise, or at least don't use often. Beyond hours of non-stop paddling, there could be lifting the watercraft, portaging, or lifting or pulling the watercraft over logs or down shallow rapids. Be in shape for the trip. To not be could result in a stranding and the need for rescue.

Anytime you are on water in any type watercraft, having and using an approved personal flotation device (PFD) is a must and a legal requirement.

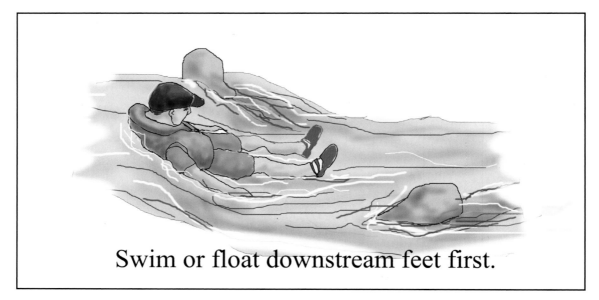

Swim or float downstream feet first.

A canoe, raft, or boat overturn in rapids requires quick thinking to protect the head from being banged on rocks. Always float feet first to give the head protection, plus this allows the survivor to see where he needs to go.

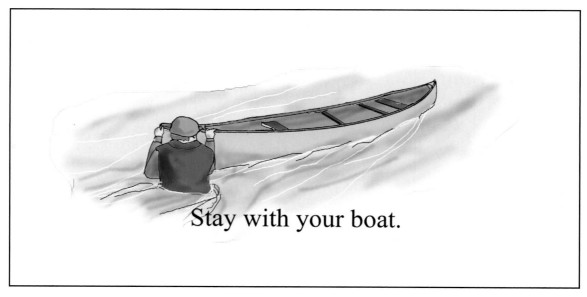

Stay with your boat.

In a boat, canoe, or raft overturn on a large lake or ocean, if the watercraft doesn't sink, stay with the floating platform as it is much easier for rescue spotters to see the watercraft than a person floating in a large body of water.

For float trips on creeks, rivers, and lakes, having extra paddles can be a lifesaver. If a motor is used, then spare parts and a tool kit are a must, as is a fire extinguisher. All water craft should have a repair kit suitable for that craft onboard and a member of the group who has the mechanical skills to make repairs. I was on a several-weeks-long remote canoe trip in northern Canada when a roll of duct tape allowed me to repair a hole in my canoe and the trip continued; otherwise I would have been stranded.

If you plan to take a trip out into a large body of water such as an ocean, bay, or sprawling inland lake, make sure that the boat you take is of a size and design to match the conditions that may be met on the trip. Boats of this size should have modern navigational aids, two-way radios capable of talking to the Coast Guard, and a seasoned boat pilot. Large open water can become dangerous in just minutes from sudden weather changes, an equipment failure, or accident such as a fire on board. Use caution when planning a trip of this type and get the best boat and crew for the conditions. Study ocean survival before you take such a trip. If the water is cold where you plan your ocean trip, be sure the boat is equipped with survival suits and that you know how to get into one and use it correctly. In cold water, they are a must.

If your float trip involves a boat with a motor, make sure you take enough fuel. The Coast Guard will tell you that many boaters get into trouble both on ocean trips and in large backcountry lakes simply because they run out of fuel. Be sure the tanks of the boat you are in are full before leaving the dock. Don't take a trip so long that you can't reach your destination on a third of a tank. Plan on a third going out, a third returning, and a third in reserve for emergencies.

Trips on small streams and lakes should start with each person having a personal flotation device (PFD) and knowing how to float in it to slow hypothermia. Most survival situations in this environment start with a capsized watercraft and everyone in the water. If rapids are part of the trip, then they need to know that if the craft has been overturned or sunk, they need to go down rapids feet-first with their legs acting as shock absorbers as they hit rocks.

On large lakes where the shore may be too far away to swim to, assuming the watercraft doesn't sink, stay with the craft as it is much easier for searchers to spot you hanging onto the craft by searchers and it doesn't take as much energy if you hang onto the side of the craft.

Also each person on the trip needs to have a survival kit attached to them because as soon as they make the shore the basics of wilderness survival kick in. Be sure to set up your survival camp near the shore as that will be the first place search and rescue will be looking.

Finally, do not forget that the one of the most common causes of small watercraft accidents is overloading. Never take on more passengers than the watercraft is designed to hold.

SWAMPS

The word "swamp" means many things to many people. To some, it is a forbidding, wet environment that humans should avoid at all costs. To others, it is an adventurous place rich in scenery, nature, game, and fish, a locale where peace of mind comes easy.

Webster's Dictionary defines swamp as "wet spongy land saturated and sometimes partially or intermittently covered with water." The US Department of the Interior's Fish and Wildlife Service has an official definition: "Swamp is all wetlands with greater than 50 percent of its area in cover of woody plants; that is, trees, brush, vines, etc."

A typical peat bog.

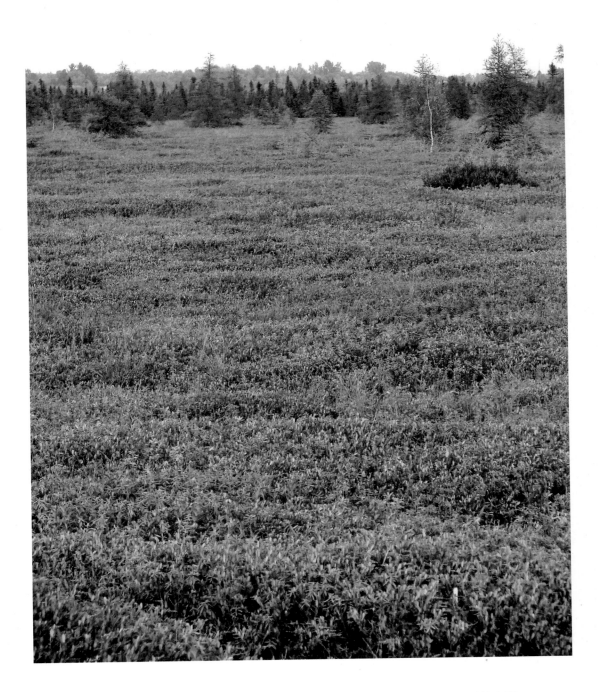

THE SCOUT'S GUIDE TO WILDERNESS SURVIVAL AND FIRST AID

Many people confuse marshlands with swamps. Marshes are almost totally devoid of any bushes or trees. Most marshes are created by tidal activity, and they are usually in areas with high saline or alkaline content in the soil. Marshes are usually covered in grass-like plants and are usually associated with the ocean.

Other people mistake bogs for swamps. Bogs are usually the remains of ancient lakes. While swamps have a covering of trees and woody plants, bogs are covered with mosses, ferns, and lichens. Until you step in a bog, you usually don't see the water. Then the bog acts like a wet sponge.

There are swamps in almost every region of North America. This comes as a surprise to many people who normally think of swamps as something found only in the Deep South.

The origins of swamps are varied. Many are the result of centuries of change in river flows. Swamps along the Mississippi River and the Ohio River were formed this way. Some swamps are the result of glacial activities—swamps in Canada, around the Great Lakes, and in New England are of this type. Still other swamps were created by falling meteorites, such as the Carolina Bays; by receding ocean, such as the Okefenokee Swamp; or by an earthquake, such as Reelfoot Swamp. Today new swamps are being created at a rapid rate by the activity of beavers. There seem to be almost as many ways that swamps are created as there, are swamps.

When you begin to consider exploring, hunting, fishing, camping, canoeing, or trapping in the swamps, you may be surprised at how much negative feedback you will hear about swamps in general. For centuries, Americans have been kept out of nature-rich swamps by horror tales and negative folklore. Quicksand . . . black panthers . . . snakes . . . spiders . . . alligators . . . lost! These associations and others have been too often connected with swamps. Television and movies have capitalized on these fears in misleading movies filmed in so-called swamp settings.

Historians tell us that this fear of swamps came about during the early exploration of North America. Since there are few swamps in Europe, the European explorers avoided swamps. Lack of experience with this new swamp environment made them mysterious to explorers. Native Americans were quick to recognize white men's fear of swamps and told them frightening stories to keep the swamps to   themselves. With the passing of each generation these swamp stories grew and were handed down as fact. We still have many swamp phobias with us today that are the result of centuries-old tales.

Swamps are among our last wilderness areas, and many of them offer a backcountry setting near urban areas. Because of the fear and ignorance so many people have of swamps, there are still many swamps scattered over North America that remain totally wild. These swamps serve many beneficial purposes and we are fortunate that we have them. They are the last preserves for many of our endangered plants and animals. They are also great water storage areas and are constantly recharging underground water supplies. The trees and lush plants in swamps help keep us in oxygen.

Of equal importance is the swamp's role in providing recreation and adventure. Swamps are excellent fauna and flora habitats; nowhere will you find better hunting and fishing. Because swamps are rich in suitable wildlife habitat and have suffered less from the pressures of progress than any other parts of the American landscape, they constitute the outdoorsman's last paradise. At the same time, swamps may suddenly require survival skills.

Why Are Swamps Difficult?

Because a swamp is a wet environment in which there are few roads and thick vegetation, it can put you in a survival predicament quickly. Basically, there are three common swamp predicaments that are dangerous.

1. With the debris typical in swamp water, it is easy to foul an outboard motor or to puncture a canoe, kayak, inflatable raft; or for a four-wheel-drive vehicle to become hopelessly stuck in the always unpredictable mud and muck.
2. It is easy to get lost. Since swamp terrain is generally flat, everything tends to look alike on an overcast day. Much of the vegetation in the swamp looks the same, and landmarks are often near impossible to establish or recognize.
3. You or a group member could become sick or injured and not be able to get help. Strandings in swamps are often difficult to avoid. A top priority when you go into a swamp should always be to let someone know where you are going and when you plan to return. File a trip plan. Always keep your equipment in good repair and have a back-up system or at least a repair kit that you know how to use. Avoid weather that could get you into trouble, and avoid areas from which your return may be impossible In other words, anytime you are venturing into a swamp, use common sense.

No one should ever go into a swamp alone. Be sure to let your group know generally where you plan to explore, hunt, fish, or hike, and when you plan to return. Also tell someone at your home, motel, or lodge where you are going and when you plan to return.

An extra precaution is to leave a note on the windshield of your car stating your name, the direction in which you are traveling, and when you plan to return. While these basic rules, which I emphasize many times in this book, can't prevent you from having an immobilizing accident, they can cut down on the number of hours your ordeal lasts.

Swamps are also difficult because they are watery environments, and travel in a straight line is usually impossible for any great distance. Following the known water course across the swamp often defies most navigational principles. In most cases, a local guide who is familiar with the swamp is a must if you are to go from one point to another in a reasonable amount of time.

Swamp Survival Techniques

Techniques for surviving in a swamp are very similar to techniques discussed throughout this book. However, there are a few points peculiar to swamp survival that should be emphasized.

Making it easier to be found.

Once you realize that you are lost in a swamp, the very first thing you need to do is to stop. A swamp is no place to be wandering about. The same thing applies if you are stranded, as by a hole in your kayak or canoe, or an outboard motor which has stopped. Don't attempt to walk out. Stay where you are, or move only a short distance to get into a more open area where you may be spotted easily from the air.

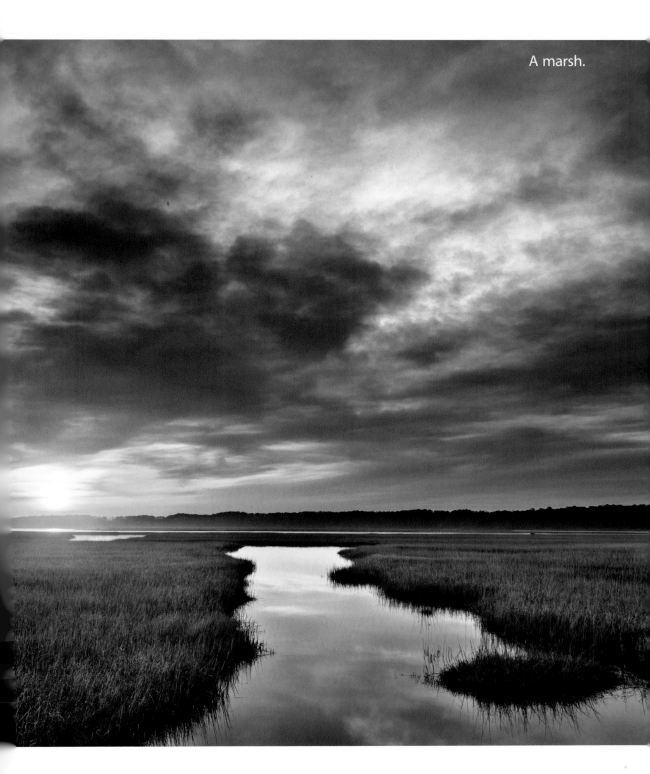

A marsh.

The importance of an opening cannot be overemphasized in the case of a swamp. Many times I have been looking in a swamp for someone who was lost and had a canoe or boat with him. Because of the lush overhead vegetation, I have flown over such people without ever seeing them.

If you have a boat or canoe, try to secure it where it can be seen from overhead. Once you have an opening in which to await rescue, use some sort of signal so that you will be more easily spotted. Review Chapter 9 in this book on signaling. Also use your imagination. However, many times in the case of a boat or canoe, once it is in the opening, it is easily spotted from the air, especially if those who are searching for you know that you were traveling by boat or canoe.

Protection from the elements.

Once you have established an opening in which to await rescue, the first thing to consider is what protections are necessary. During cool or cold weather in a swamp, hypothermia is one of the first concerns, being in a wet environment, being tired, being scared, all go together to bring on hypothermia. As quickly as possible, build a fire. Even in this wet environment, a fire can be started by following the techniques discussed in Chapter 8.

Obviously, if you have to await rescue in a boat because getting on dry land is impossible or not practical, bundle up as much as you can to prevent hypothermia. Consider putting on raingear to cut the chilling effect of the wind.

If you are caught in a swamp during warm weather, your immediate attention may be directed to protection from mosquitoes and blackflies. These biting insects are just as dangerous as, if not more dangerous than, any snakes or other critters you are likely to run into in the swamps. Take plenty of insect repellent with you and long sleeve shirt and long pants.

Lightning is another danger during warm weather. As an example of how terrifying lightning can be, several years ago I was guiding an Ohio fisherman in a swamp in East Texas when a sudden and fierce thunderstorm hit. We were caught out in some tall timber. I asked my client to lie down in the boat and prepared to crank the motor and move into a stand of thick, low-growing brush. He was shocked that I would even think of putting the boat into that "cottonmouth-infested brush." As he was preaching to me the dangers of snakes, a bolt of lightning clobbered a nearby cypress with an earsplitting crack. Pieces of bark flew in all directions. My client dived into the bottom of the boat and begged me to get into the low-growing bushes. The storm lasted two long hours, with the severity of a mortar attack. On the way back to camp, my pale client told me that snakes were now only his second-biggest fear in the swamp—lightning was first!

Drinking water.

You'd think that the last problem you'd have in a swamp survival situation would be that of finding water. Granted, there is usually plenty of water available in most swamps, but many times the water is not safe to drink. In fact, most swamps offer few, if any, sources of safe drinking water. Many of today's swamps are fed by waters that originate upstream, and these streams may be polluted by waste from cities, industries, agricultural areas, and even rural septic tanks. Regardless of how clear the swamp water may look, don't trust it. Some swamps that are made up primarily of standing water contain stagnant water that is subject to bacteriological contamination from

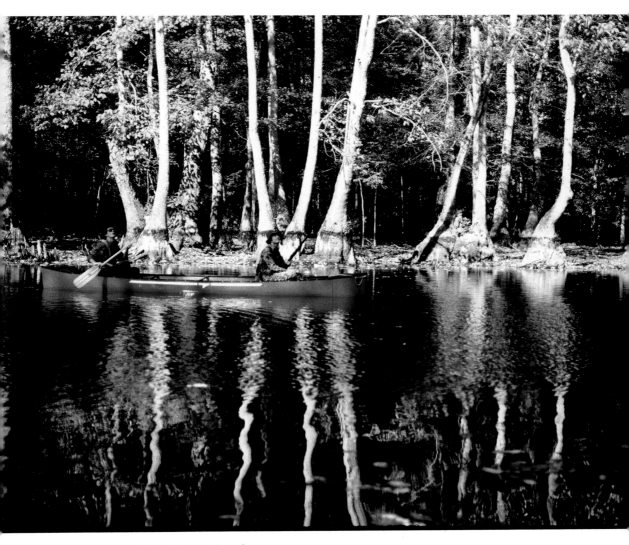

A typical swamp of the Deep South.

animals. Other swamps, such as the rapidly growing number of beaver swamps, contain populations of animals that carry a variety of potential illnesses to man.

The National Park Service states, "We know of no swamp waters that have met a safe drinking water test." It is only good judgment to purify the water regardless of how pure it may look. I can testify that this is true. Several years ago two of my friends went deep into a swamp in southern Mississippi on a week-long search for bull bluegills. The running water next to their camp looked so clean that they didn't bother to treat it. That was a mistake that cut their trip short. They were weeks getting their digestive systems back into proper working order.

Needless to say, if you're dying of thirst, the long-range effect of drinking contaminated water is something you will have to worry about later. However, if it is at all possible to treat the water you are going to drink, you should do so. Chapter 10 in this book concerning drinking water is very important. With the modern methods of treating water, there is no excuse for not having good water to drink while you are in the swamp, even in a survival situation. Think ahead. If your swamp trip takes you far from treated water, go prepared. Take enough water with you and take along a method of treating the water.

Gear for swamp survival is very similar to survival gear for other areas. Many times in southern swamps, I have used the same survival kit that I use in the Arctic. However, also be sure to have insect repellent, a good supply of waterproof matches, and, if possible, a machete. The machete is one of the best survival knives in a swamp environment. It can do much to make your stay more comfortable. It can be used for everything from simple camp chores to opening up a clearing where you can be seen from' overhead.

The person who finds him- or herself stranded or lost in a swamp has little to fear, provided he has filed a trip plan and carries a survival kit with him. Many of the fears associated with swamps are unfounded.

18

WHEN A MEMBER OF YOUR GROUP IS MISSING

Have you been on an outing when you suddenly realized you were lost or stranded, unable to return to camp or your vehicle? If not, get ready, because if you go into the backcountry enough, chances are it will happen eventually. As a wildlife professional, I have spent considerable time looking for missing people in the outdoors. Most of the time, they are simply turned around in the woods and are easily found.

However, some are injured and unable to move, often due to a fall. Once, a guide who worked for me fell into an abandoned well.

Unfortunately, some outdoor enthusiasts are brought out dead as a result of heart attacks, falls, or hypothermia. The cause of death is often brought on by the stress of being lost.

While many outdoor people are learning what to do if they should become lost or stranded, few know what to do if their buddy does not make it back to the car or camp when he or she is supposed to. Every group, be it an outing club or just two friends, should plan ahead for that moment when one of them is missing. This is just as important if you are exploring on your own back forty as in a remote wilderness.

It should be a policy that every member of the group let the others know specifically where he is going and when he plans to return. All members of the group should agree to sit tight once they realize they are lost. This should be stressed over and over again. Every member of the group should carry a compass (that they know how to use), a GPS, a map of the area, cell phone, a knife, and a survival kit.

Know the medical condition of your companions. If a member of your group has a heart problem, seizures, or other medical problem, make sure a buddy goes with him. An unconscious person needs to be found quickly, but is extremely difficult to find.

Each member of your group needs to know how to locate the nearest conservation officer, forest ranger, or sheriff's office. In most counties in the US, the local sheriff is responsible for search and rescue. Everyone should carry the phone numbers of these officials. Delay in getting trained search-and-rescue help can be deadly.

Always be aware of how your fellow companions are dressed, what type boots they wear, and the state of mind they are in. This information is extremely valuable to search officials.

The most crucial time during a missing-buddy crisis is when you first realize that he or she is late coming into camp or back on the trail and you get no answers to your signals. Don't panic. The first rule is to stay calm and think. In most cases, lost or stranded situations are merely a sobering two- or three-hour adventure.

Signaling is an important part of the early search, as rescued people often state that while they were lost or stranded, they thought no one would bother to look for them. Select a logical point, such as where he or she was last seen, the logging road or field nearest the "most likely" area, camp, or vehicle, and blow an automobile horn or whistle. Either of these signals is an indication to the missing person that someone is looking for him. If he is nearby, he can walk to the sound. For this reason, it is crucial to blow the horn or whistle in bursts of three so that it is obviously a signal and not some unrelated noise. Pause between bursts of three and listen carefully for a reply. If the missing person has a whistle, and he should, you may hear a response immediately. If you are getting no response to your initial signaling, and feel that your buddy may be in trouble, seek out a forest ranger, conservation officer, or sheriff's department official to get trained search-and-rescue people on the scene as soon as possible. If you leave to obtain professional help, leave someone at the signal point; while one person goes for help, another should stay to continue signaling and listening.

Attempting to set up your own search is generally a bad idea, since most often untrained people with the best of intentions usually do more harm than good. They destroy valuable clues and often become lost or hurt themselves. Searching for missing people is a skill best left to those trained.

However, in some specific circumstances, such as when help is hours away or when the tract of land is not large and it is known almost exactly where the missing person is likely to be, fellow outdoorsmen might conduct a limited search. In those exceptional cases, follow these guidelines:

1. Get the entire group together to plan your search.
2. To help identify clues that you find, find out what each member knows, such as when and where the missing person was last seen, what their trip plan was, what brand of candy they eat, what type of sole do they have on their boots and their size, where they most likely went, and so on.
3. Establish someone in the group as leader of the search, and everyone does as he or she says.
4. Leave someone at the original spot to continue signaling.
5. If a specific spot is known, two searchers should begin the search with thorough examination of that immediate area in case there was a health problem or injury. Take care not to destroy any signs. It is important that only one or two do this, as a larger group will destroy clues that might be helpful if a professional search is needed.

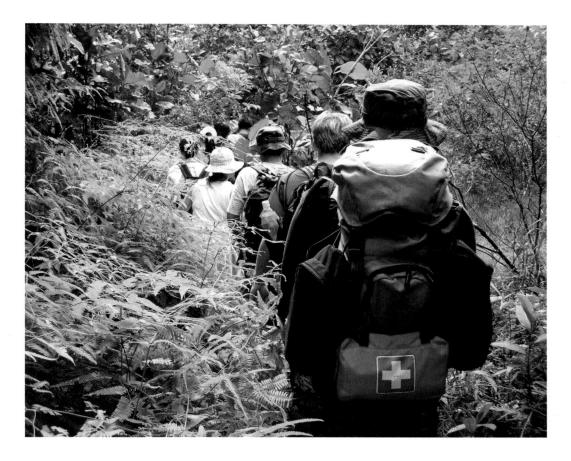

6. Look for signs, such as tracks, for an indication of the missing person's direction of travel.
7. Due to the excitement of the moment, searchers often get lost themselves, so mark the trail you take in so you can follow it out.
8. Consider what sounds the missing person can hear—farm, railroad, highway, mill whistle, etc.—and send someone to that location. Rather than sit still, many lost people will try to walk to sounds such as these.
9. If there are roads around the area, a vehicle should patrol these roads regularly, but do not blow the horn as you travel as the lost person will start in the direction of the horn, only to have it change directions. I have found lost people who would have been found quickly if they hadn't spent the night chasing the sounds of moving truck horns.
10. If there is a long opening in the area, such as railroad tracks, gas line, electric line right-of-way, or large fields, have someone watch these areas with binoculars.
11. Plan a signal or specific time for calling off the search. If the missing person has not been found within a short time, turn the search over to professionals.

If you and your outdoor companions have prepared for the day one of you is missing, chances are you will never be faced with a tragedy.

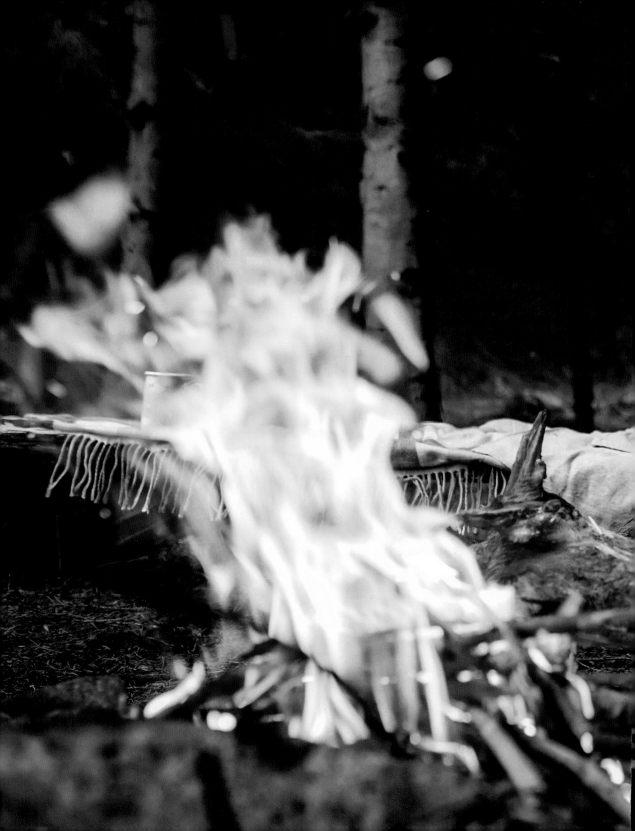

APPENDIX I

BSA REQUIREMENTS FOR THE WILDERNESS SURVIVAL MERIT BADGE:

1. Do the following:
   (a) Explain to your counselor the hazards you are most likely to encounter while participating in wilderness survival activities, and what you should do to anticipate, help prevent, mitigate, or lessen these hazards.
   (b) Show that you know first aid for and how to prevent injuries or illnesses likely to occur in backcountry settings, including hypothermia, heat reactions, frostbite, dehydration, blisters, insect stings, tick bites, and snakebites.
2. From memory list the seven priorities for survival in a backcountry or wilderness location. Explain the importance of each one with your counselor.
3. Describe ways to avoid panic and maintain a high level of morale when lost, and explain why this is important.
4. Describe the steps you would take to survive in the following exposure conditions:
   (a) Cold and snowy
   (b) Wet
   (c) Hot and dry
   (d) Windy
   (e) At or on the water
5. Put together a personal survival kit and be able to explain how each item in it could be useful.
6. Using three different methods (other than matches), build and light three fires.
7. Do the following:
   (a) Show five different ways to attract attention when lost.
   (b) Demonstrate how to use a signal mirror.
   (c) Describe from memory five ground-to-air signals and tell what they mean.
8. Improvise a natural shelter. For the purpose of this demonstration, use techniques that have little negative impact on the environment. Spend a night in your shelter.
9. Explain how to protect yourself from insects, reptiles, bears, and other animals of the local region.
10. Demonstrate three ways to treat water found in the outdoors to prepare it for drinking.

11. Show that you know the proper clothing to wear while in the outdoors during extremely hot and cold weather and during wet conditions.
12. Explain why it usually is not wise to eat edible wild plants or wildlife in a wilderness survival situation.

APPENDIX II

WEB ADDRESSES FOR SURVIVAL PRODUCTS MENTIONED IN THIS BOOK

Adventure Medical Kits – www.adventuremedicalkits.com
After Bite/After Burn – www.afterbite.com
BugX Insect Repellent – www.coretexproducts.com
Coghlan's Tube Tent – www.coghlans.com
FireSteel Magnesium Rod – www.firesteel.com
Fox 40 Whistle – www.fox40world.com
LifeStraw Water Filter – www.lifestraw.com
MRC Medical Emergency Sleeping Bag – www.mrcmedical.com
Potable Aqua Water Treatment Tablets – www.potableaqua.com
Sawyer Water Filter – www.sawyer.com
Spot Personal Locator Beacon – www.findmespot.com
StarFlash Signal Mirror – www.ultimatesurvival.com
SureFire Flashlights – www.surefire.com
ThermaCell Insect Repellent – www.thermacell.com
WindStorm Whistle – www.stormwhistles.com

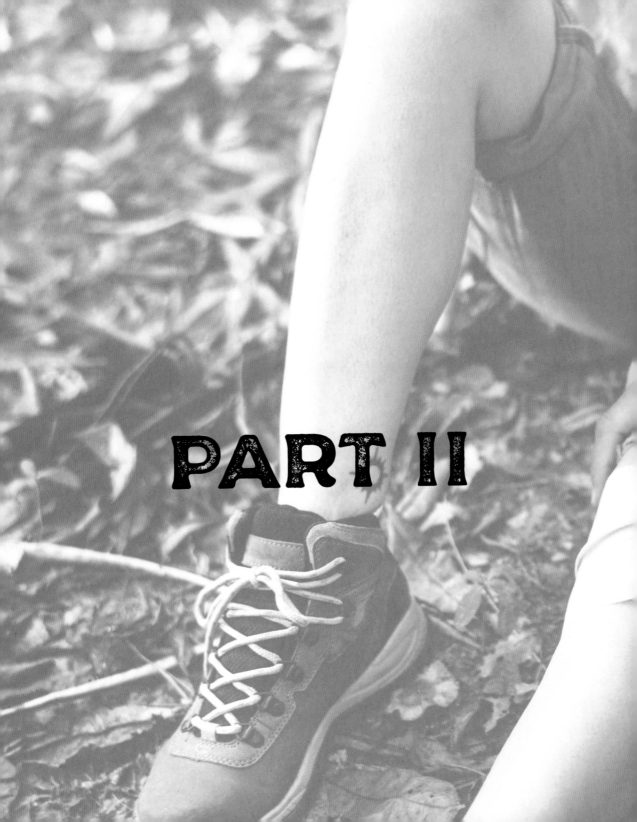

PART II

FIRST AID

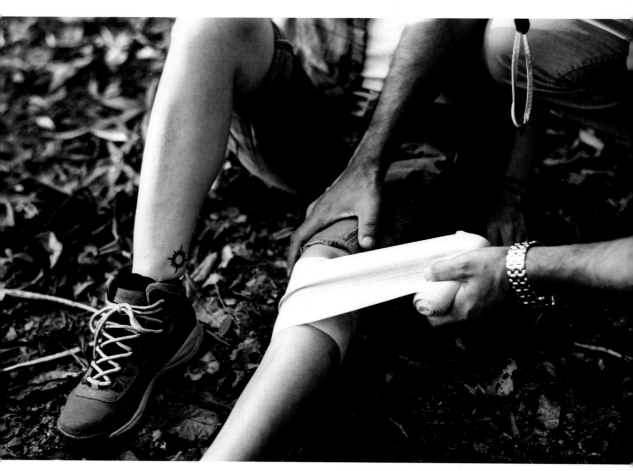

An in-depth knowledge of wilderness first aid can come in handy.

INTRODUCTION

Five years ago I published the *Wilderness First Aid Handbook*. That book was the culmination of several years of discussions with students, instructors, and educators while serving as Medical Advisor for Stanford Outdoor Education. I had wanted to provide protocols that could deliver logical and useful guidance for first responders whose depth of medical knowledge was a sixteen-hour wilderness first aid (WFA) course. I attempted to stay within the bounds of the curriculum and course that have been adopted and taught throughout the United States. In preparation for this Scouting edition, I revisited the doctrine and the evidence that forms the backbone of wilderness first aid, and remembered the lessons (delivered and received) over the years from my emergency medicine residents and wilderness medicine fellows in the Stanford

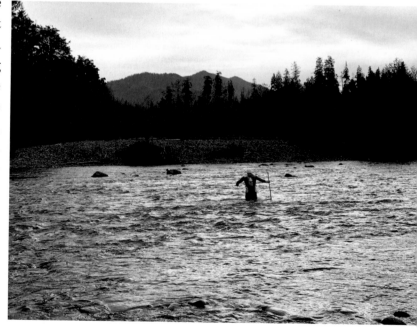

Before going on a trip in the wilderness, consider taking a first-aid course. *Credit: Grant Lipman*

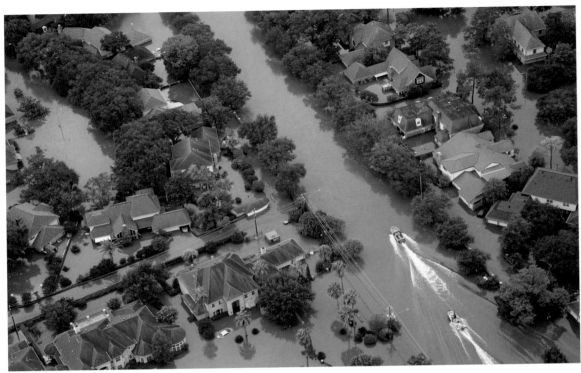

Wilderness first aid skills may come in handy in areas affected by natural disasters.

Department of Emergency Medicine. I decided to expand the scope of this edition to reflect both the WFA core curriculum as well as complex concepts and skills, as often readers have a thirst for advanced knowledge.

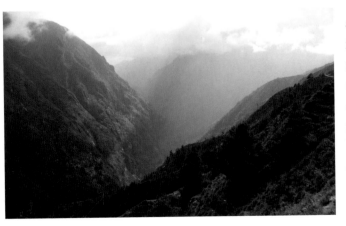

Wilderness first aid is the assessment and treatment of an ill or injured person in an environment where definitive medical care by a professional or rapid transport to definitive care is unavailable. People who work, live, travel, and recreate in the outdoors have special-

Wilderness first aid courses can prepare you for when you're the first person on the scene. *Credit: Grant Lipman*

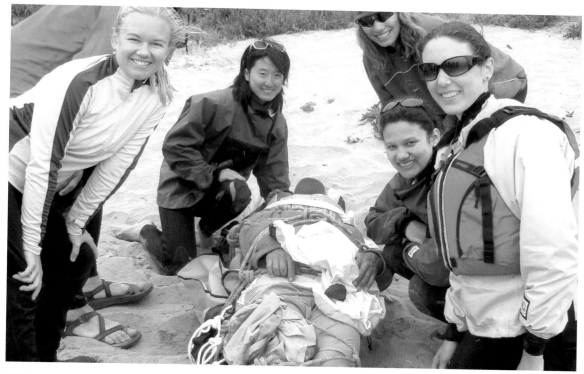

Wilderness first aid courses can teach you how to assess an ill or injured individual.
Credit: Grant Lipman

ized medical needs not adequately fulfilled by traditional first aid. Wilderness first aid fills this gap. Remote locations, arduous conditions, paucity of diagnostic and therapeutic equipment, and a need to make critical decisions, often without outside communication, define wilderness medicine as a specialty. These conditions may be found in remote wilderness, the developing world, or even in wealthy urban areas beset by natural disasters. This book is to be used as a guide to aug-

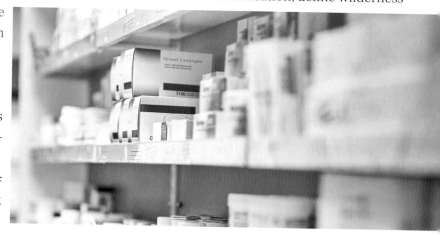

You can purchase most of the medicines in this book over the counter.

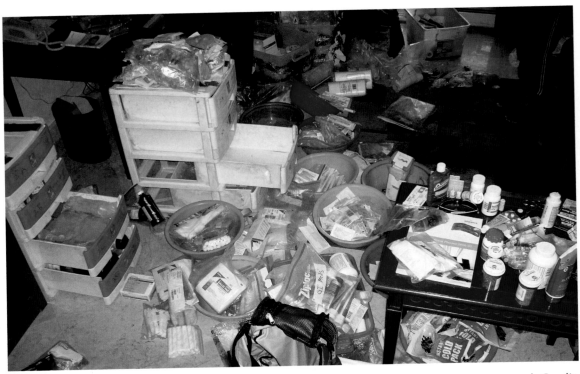

Consult with a doctor about any medicines you carry or prescriptions you may need. *Credit: Grant Lipman*

ment the skills and training learned in a typical wilderness first aid course. The intention is to assist the lay public, outdoor professionals, and instructors as well as members of wilderness first aid classes with useful and practical information that complements their training. Some elective skills are included, which the individual can decide to include depending on his or her comfort level and specific training.

This book is written for those who have basic first aid knowledge, not necessarily those with advanced degrees in medicine or pre-hospital care. The American Heart Association has limited components of its resuscitation curriculum, recognizing that some tasks may be difficult for laypersons to competently perform. Similarly, this book acknowledges that certain knowledge and procedures are outside the scope of the average wilderness first aid provider's knowledge, and thus strives to limit the use of technical terms or advanced techniques that may be unfamiliar to some readers or impractical based on the wilderness setting. This book provides easy-to-follow protocols and instructions to assist those encountering most wilderness emergencies.

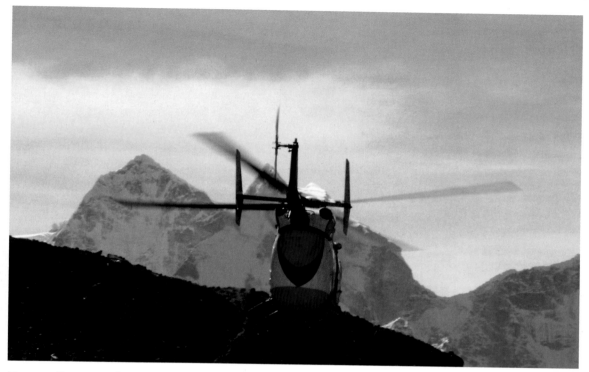

Depending on where you are in the wilderness during an emergency, medical personnel may need a boat or helicopter to reach you. *Credit: Grant Lipman*

While the contents of this book are meant to assist in managing a medical emergency in a remote environment, the information is applicable to any setting where the reader is first on the scene. The protocols contained in this book are to be used as guidelines and are by no means a substitution for common sense or definitive medical care. A rescuer is liable for his or her own actions and should never undertake a medical procedure he or she feels uncomfortable with or which is not absolutely necessary unless the rescuer believes the victim may lose their life or limb without intervention.

Most medicines discussed in this book can be purchased over the counter. Consult with a doctor concerning the potential side effects, complications, or contraindications of any medications you carry. Similarly, ensure that there are no known allergies to the medicines you use.

Travel in the wilderness is an inherently risky activity, as one often travels to remote locations for the adventure, solitude, and serenity provided. Ultimately, the ethos of self-reliance found in the backcountry is epitomized by a wilderness medical emergency. These protocols assume knowledge and implementation of patient assessment systems that should not be ignored when acting on these protocols. Familiarize yourself with the information within these pages before venturing into the backcountry to minimize the chances that an accident will have to be an emergency.

This danger symbol next to the "red flags" of a patient's symptoms serves as an indicator of a dangerous disease process that may necessitate imminent evacuation to definitive medical care. If any of these "red flags" are observed, start early preparations for a potential evacuation. Consideration of the terrain, time of day, and weather are all potential issues in expediting a timely evacuation.

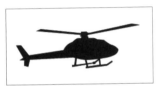

This helicopter symbol next to the "evacuate" assumes a medical emergency that requires a higher level of care via Emergency Medical Services (EMS). All evacuations assume the emergency is taking place in a setting where communication is likely not possible. The severity of the emergency, the potential for the patient to decompensate, the availability (or lack thereof) of outside communication, and the logistical and timely constraints of a rescue versus self-evacuation all need to be taken into consideration. **If patients are able to ambulate on their own without endangering themselves or others, self-evacuation may be a quicker and better option in the wilderness environment.** If a victim is unable to walk, or you expect that the ability to ambulate may shortly become compromised, you should likely send for a rescue. If the decision is made to send a messenger to initiate an EMS rescue, two people (buddy system) are better than one to ensure the safe delivery of both the message and messengers.

> If the reader of this book is unsure of the necessity of an evacuation, they should likely err on the side of caution. "When in doubt, get out."

1

ASSESSMENT SYSTEM/CPR

Before you are able to administer first aid, an assessment must be made in an orderly process to ensure that both the rescuer and the patient are kept safe. Providing aid for a traumatic injury is similar to considering the causes of a sickness or random pains. The processes are the same, and a systematic approach to the problem will allow a logical step-by-step assessment, stabilization, and treatment. In the setting of trauma, rushing to provide care without an orderly

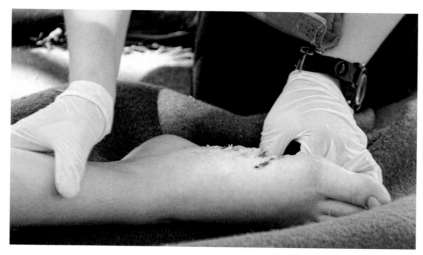

If you have gloves on the scene of the emergency, use them to protect both you and the patient.

assessment of the scene may inadvertently turn the rescuer into a victim. Keep in mind the adage, "Don't just stand there, do something." The initial assessment should consider hazards that could cause immediate injuries to the people attempting to assist the injured person.

SCENE SIZE-UP

- Ensure it is safe for the rescuer to approach the patient.
- Consider the number of patients.
- Consider the mechanism of injury (MOI), or how the patient may have been injured and the need for immediate spine immobilization (*see* Trauma).
- If body substances are present, consider gloves or eye protection precaution in order to protect both you and the patient.

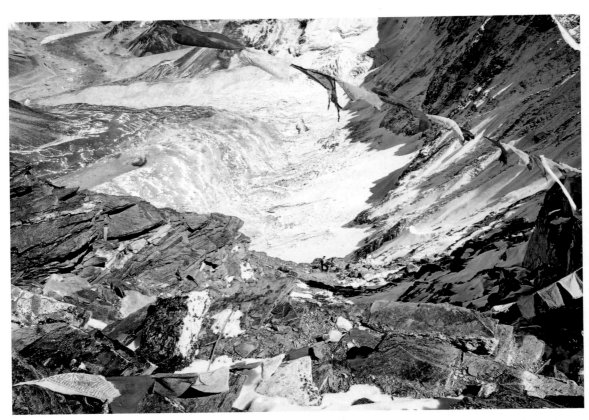

Ensure the scene is safe for the rescuer prior to approaching a potential patient.
Credit: Grant Lipman

PRIMARY ASSESSMENT

After the scene has been assessed and you are certain it is safe to approach the patient, the next step is to identify immediate threats to life. If a problem is found, stop and fix it before moving on. The primary assessment should identify potential causes of death, including lack of oxygen from a blocked airway or inadequate breathing, loss of circulation from bleeding (either internal or external) or inadequate pumping from the heart, damage to the brain or spinal cord, or extremes of the environment or metabolism. If there is a patient who has a decreased level of responsiveness (LOR) and cannot respond, you may need to use your CPR training. If multiple victims are encountered, assessing the entire scene and determining where you can do the most good to the most people should dictate your priority. For example, you may need to apply a tourniquet to a heavily bleeding limb before you check the breathing on a non-responsive person.

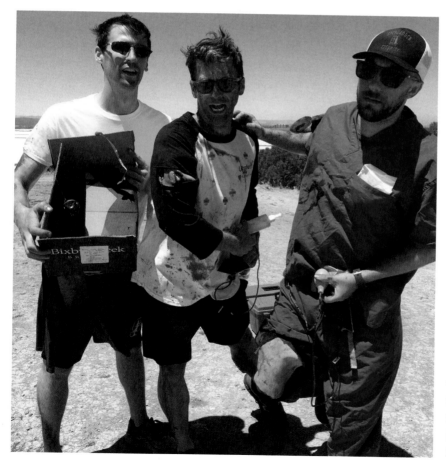

It may be necessary to control the bleeding to an injured limb prior to checking the breathing. *Credit: Grant Lipman*

Primary Assessment Procedure

- Introduce and identify yourself as you approach the patient.
- Obtain verbal consent to treat them.
- Establish responsiveness.
- Level of responsiveness (LOR): A-V-P-U—Alert, Verbal, Pain, Unresponsive.

ABCDE

- **A**irway
  - ➢ Check the patient's airway.
  - ➢ If a patient can talk, he or she has an open airway.
  - ➢ If necessary, open the airway by the head tilt/chin lift.

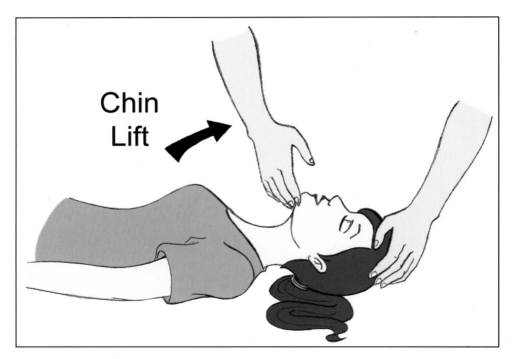

Head tilt/chin lift.

  - ➢ Look in the mouth to clear any obstructions.
  - ➢ Heimlich maneuver/abdominal thrusts if the person appears to be choking or if there is an obstructing foreign body.

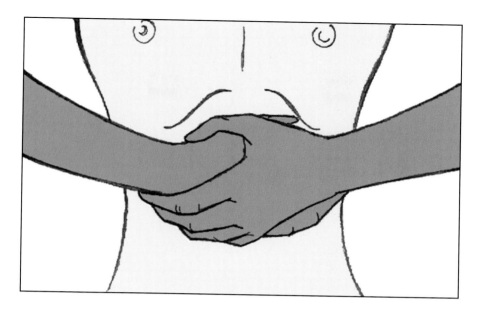

Hands position for Heimlich maneuver.

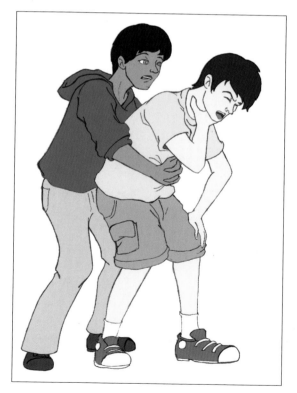

Heimlich maneuver.

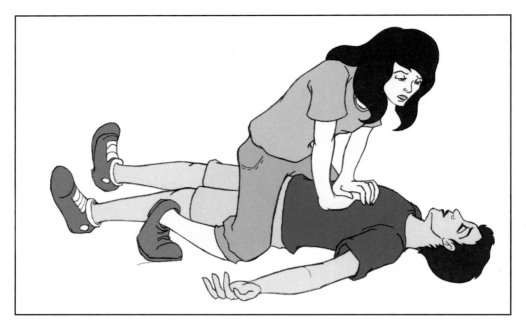

Abdominal thrusts for an unconscious choking victim.

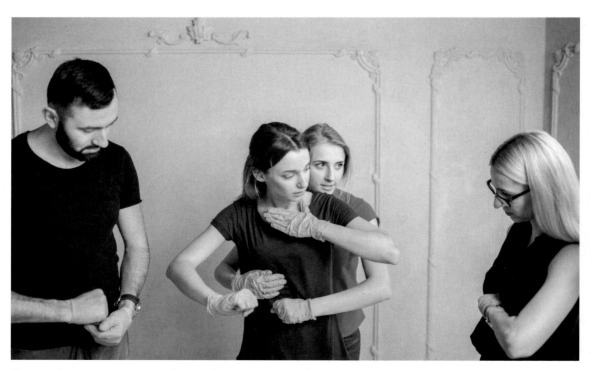

First aid courses can teach you how to properly give the Heimlich maneuver.

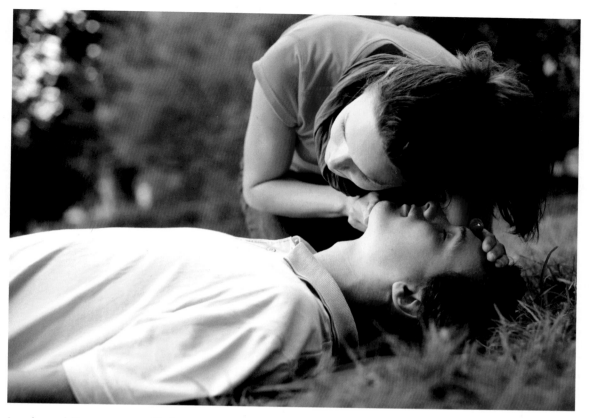

Look and listen to see if the patient is breathing. If they aren't, proceed to CPR.

- **B**reathing
  - ➢ Look and listen for breathing.
  - ➢ No breathing? (*see* CPR).
  - ➢ Assess if the breathing is difficult or painful (*see* Chest Pain, Chest Trauma, and/or Lung Problems).
- **C**irculation
  - ➢ Check to see if there is obvious major bleeding.
  - ➢ If massive bleeding or rapid pulse, check for site of bleeding and take appropriate action through either direct pressure or application of a tourniquet (*see* Wound Care).
  - ➢ Feel for a pulse.
  - ➢ No pulse? (*see* CPR)

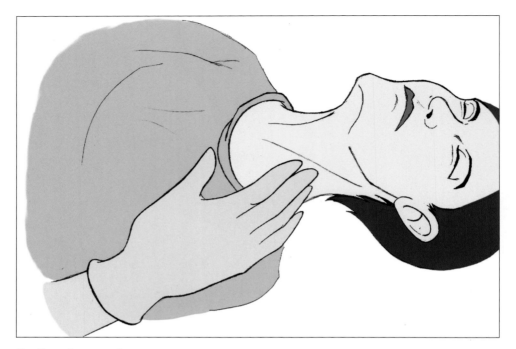

Feeling for a pulse.

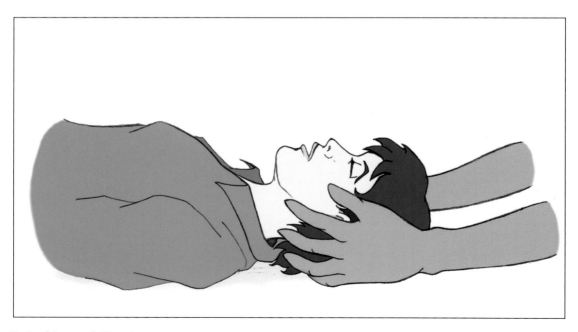

Spinal immobilization.

- **D**ecide/**D**isability
  - ➤ Consider the MOI and decide early if there is a necessity for spinal immobilization and control the head (*see* Trauma).
- **E**xposure/**E**nvironment
  - ➤ Expose serious wounds for full evaluation and treatment. Consider environmental causes (heat, cold, lightning) for the injury or illness as well as protecting the patient from further environmental stressors as treatment progresses (i.e., place on an insulating pad sooner rather than later in the care).

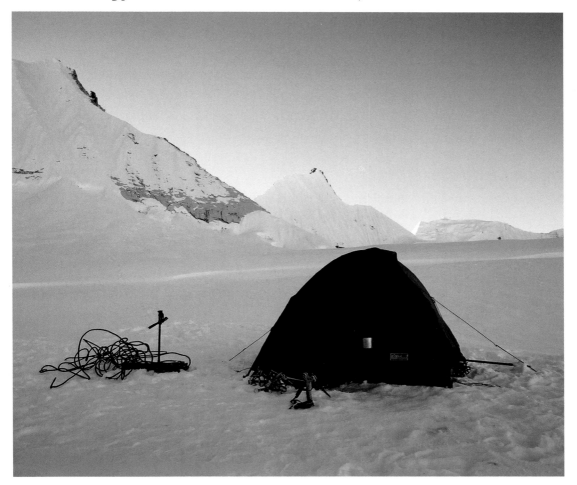

Consider possible environmental causes, such as cold temperature, for the patient's injury. *Credit: Grant Lipman*

SECONDARY ASSESSMENT

Once evaluation of any immediate life-threatening events is complete, you are ready to perform a comprehensive and focused assessment of the injury and illness. This will involve gathering a complete history and performing a thorough physical exam from head to toe in a systematic manner. The initial survey should have found and corrected immediate critical conditions; the secondary assessment will now determine if other less obvious injuries can be identified. For example, a broken bone is painful and may be a distraction to both the patient and rescuer, but may make a rescuer overlook other more serious injuries.

The secondary assessment should be thorough, with direct and simple questions. Pushing everywhere may elicit subtle areas of tenderness. Sliding a hand under a shirt may find a hidden area of blood loss. The outcome of this secondary assessment will lead to system specific protocols and decisions for treatment and/or evacuation to definitive medical care. Most methodologic approaches start at the head and work down towards the feet. Always let the patient know what you are doing and where you are about to touch so they are not alarmed or offended. While performing the secondary survey, move the patient as little as possible to avoid aggravating any injuries.

Secondary Assessment Procedure

- Determine the chief complaint (what hurts or is bothering the patient).
- History of the illness (when and how it happened).
- **SAMPLE** History:
  - ➢ Symptoms.
  - ➢ Allergies (to medications/latex).
  - ➢ Medications.
  - ➢ Pertinent medical history.
  - ➢ Last food or drink.
  - ➢ Events that happened which may be relevant to the chief complaint.
- Check vital signs: heart rate, respiratory rate.

Physical Exam

Ask the patient where it hurts, and then, when feeling gently, ask if it hurts to be touched there. You may need to remove clothing to completely visualize the injury.

- Head. Feel the skull for swelling and depressions, look for drainage from the ears, nose, and mouth. Have the patient feel their teeth to ensure they match up, and can open and close their jaw naturally and without pain.

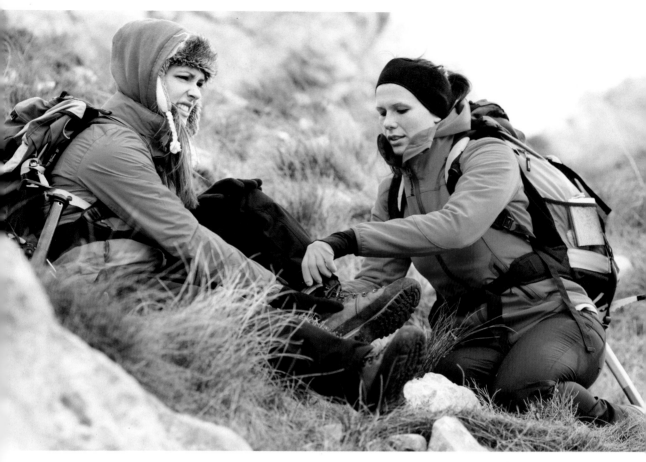

A physical exam will help you get a better idea of how to treat the patient's injury.

- Neck. Differentiate midline spinal tenderness from non-midline tense muscles and tenderness.
- Chest. Press on both sides of the chest, listen, and feel for abnormal sounds.
- Abdomen. Press on all quadrants to differentiate pain from tenderness.
- Pelvis. Gently push on the bony prominences of the pelvis at the hips.
- Legs. Feel and look for symmetry and full range of movement.
- Arms. Feel and look for symmetry and full range of movement. Press on one arm at a time, and be sure to check wrists, hands, and fingers.
- Back. Press on every bone from the top to the bottom of the spine. Consider log-roll precautions if you suspect a spinal injury.

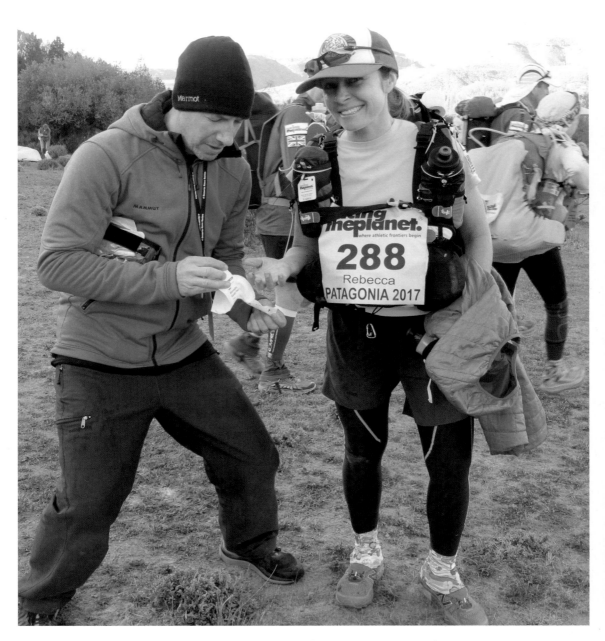

After helping your patient, make sure to document as much information as you can as soon as possible. *Credit: Grant Lipman*

The SOAP Note

Collect information and write it down as soon as possible. Document what you do and any changes to the patient. This is important for both patient care and to protect the first-aid responder. If the patient requires evacuation, the SOAP note will allow for a continuation of care and concise communication of the events that transpired in the pre-hospital setting.

- **S**ubjective/**S**ummary of the patient's age, complaints, and occurrences.
- **O**bjective/**O**bservations of the patient, vital signs, and SAMPLE history.
- **A**ssessments of what you think is wrong, and assess any changes to the patient and what may develop or change.
- **P**lan what you are going to do, and whether the patient needs an intervention or evacuation.

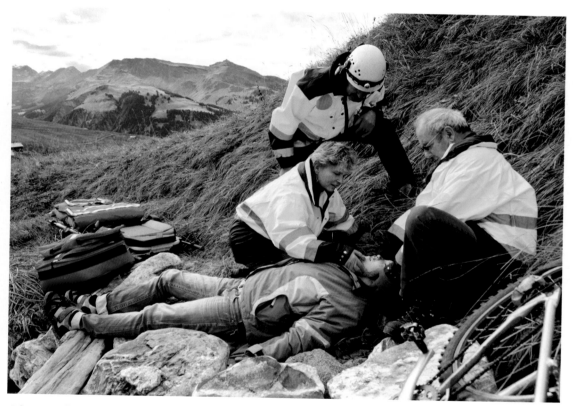

After evaluating the patient, determine whether or not they need an evacuation.

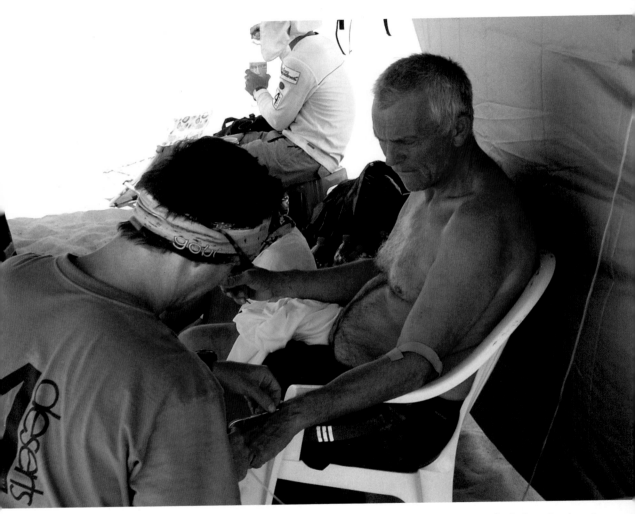

A careful history and physical can help determine the cause of abdominal pain.
Credit: Grant Lipman

2
ABDOMINAL PAIN

Abdominal pain is a potentially concerning although not uncommon complaint. Even in a hospital with all the resources of a laboratory, ultrasounds, and CT scans it can still be a challenging diagnosis. In a wilderness setting with no tools other than a thorough history and physical exam, care must be taken in evaluating the patient for clues that may necessitate an evacuation for a problem that may require medical or surgical intervention. While this is a challenging diagnostic problem in the backcountry, a thorough patient interview will be of great assistance in differentiating the causes. Abdominal pain can range from mild discomfort to a serious or deadly event. When performing the secondary assessment, press gently on all quadrants of the stomach with a flat open palm. The pain and exam may change over time. Pay attention for red flags and have a low index of suspicion to evacuate if symptoms progress or pain that lasts more than twenty-four hours.

Pain in the right upper quadrant of the abdomen may be from a problem with the gallbladder. Gallbladder disease is more common in overweight people over forty, also in women. The pain may initially be episodic, with an onset after eating, but may become constant and severe. There is no burning or "sour stomach" associated with gallbladder pain. If a fever is present this may represent an infected gallbladder, which is a surgical emergency and necessitates intravenous antibiotics and evacuation.

Pain in the right lower quadrant raises the possibility of appendicitis. This can occur in any age range. The pain typically starts arounds the belly button and then the discomfort migrates to the right lower quadrant, halfway between the belly button and top of the right hip bone. Ask

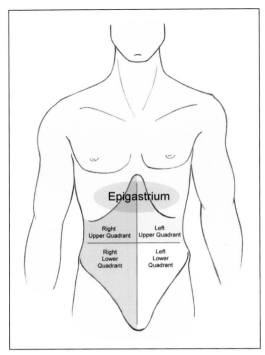

Abdomen schematic.

questions specifically to elicit when and where the pain started, and where it is now. The localization of pain and tenderness to the right lower quadrant should raise the suspicion of acute appendicitis. It may present with diarrhea and/or vomiting. Presence of this pain with a fever, increased pain with movement or pushing on other areas of the abdomen all should raise concern for a surgical emergency and evacuation. However, if someone with abdominal pain can walk comfortably and jump up and down with no discomfort, this should be reassuring that it is less likely acute appendicitis.

Left lower quadrant abdominal pain can be from diverticulitis, an infection of small outpouchings of the large bowel. This is more common in the middle-aged and elderly, and usually presents with constant, dull, and worsening pain. It can present with diarrhea, but unlike the crampy abdominal pain often found with diarrhea, this pain is localized to the left lower quadrant and reproducible with palpation. As this infection progresses, a fever usually occurs and evacuation to a hospital is needed with intravenous antibiotics and sometimes even surgery.

Diarrhea is the passage of loose or watery stools. It can be very common on trips, especially when there is poor hygiene. The watery bowel movements may present with crampy abdominal pain, sweats, malaise and fatigue, exhaustion, nausea and/or vomiting, and fevers and chills. The diarrhea can range from a mild nuisance to total debilitation. If proper hygiene is not maintained, diarrhea can easily spread through a camp, affecting lots of people. Most diarrhea while traveling is caused by ingested bacteria, and can be prevented by hand washing and water treatment. Water should be boiled, treated, or filtered before ingesting. Food should be peeled and hands washed or sanitized before eating and after having a bowel movement. Diarrhea may be caused by viruses, which are notorious for spreading among members of an outing, and while self-limited, may make life miserable for several days. Proper latrine placement (at least two hundred meters from camp) and having a "no shoes in tent" policy can minimize the risk of spreading diarrhea-causing organisms.

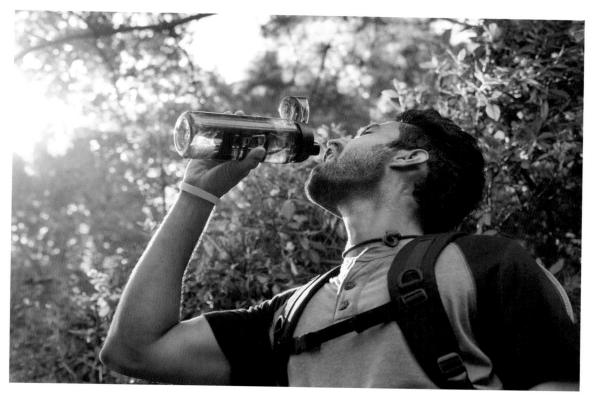

Hydrating can assist with preventing constipation.

SYMPTOMS: CONSTIPATION (NO STOOL FOR SEVERAL DAYS)

- Hard stools, bloating, distention.
- Crampy, intermittent, generalized (four quadrant) pain.
- Pain may be greater in the left lower quadrant of the abdomen.
- Patient may be doubled-over in distress.

Caffeinated drinks like coffee or tea can stimulate the bowels and lessen abdominal pain from constipation.

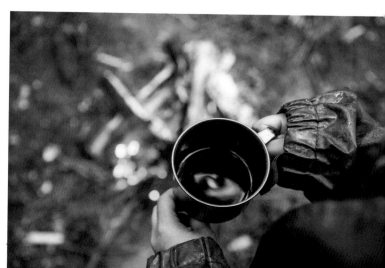

⚠️ **Red Flags:** Presence of vomiting or fever with constipation, history of small bowel obstruction, or history of abdominal surgery.

Treatment

- Maintain hydration with clear fluids.
- If dehydrated, rehydrate with electrolyte-containing fluids.
- Give caffeinated drinks (coffee, tea, hot chocolate) to stimulate the bowels.
- Give fiber or sips of mineral oil (if available).
- Give laxative (if available).
- Offer adequate latrine time.

SYMPTOMS: NAUSEA, VOMITING, DIARRHEA

- Crampy or sharp intermittent pain.
- Possibly associated with fever and/or fatigue.
- Diarrhea may be loose, watery, or with mucus.

⚠️ **Red Flags:** Diarrhea with blood, fever, or vomiting with blood.

Treatment

- Control the nausea with sips of herbal tea and Pepcid as needed (as directed by the instruction label).
- Rehydrate with electrolyte-containing solution. Start slowly (sips every five minutes), then when tolerating liquids, rehydrate until urine is clear.
- Ibuprofen or Tylenol as needed for pain (as directed by instruction label).
- If mild diarrhea (four to six stools/day), can treat with Pepto-Bismol (as directed by instruction label).
- If frequent diarrhea (six or more stools/day but no fever or blood in stool), treat with Imodium (as directed by instruction label).

SYMPTOMS: LOWER ABDOMINAL PAIN IN A FEMALE

- May be a dull or sharp pain, constant or intermittent, and may be one sided.
- May include vaginal bleeding.

⚠️ **Red Flags:** History of missed or irregular menstrual period, atypical from regular menstrual pain, one-sided pain.

Treatment

- Ibuprofen (as directed by instruction label).
- Pregnancy test.

SYMPTOMS: EPIGASTRIC PAIN OR "SOUR STOMACH"

- Pain at the top of the abdomen, may be burning, radiating up into chest or neck.
- Eating food or lying flat may worsen pain. Intermittent generalized cramping is common.

⚠ **Red Flags:** Black tarry stools, bloody stools, fever, history of peptic ulcer disease, or history of heart disease.

Treatment

- Pepcid or Pepto-Bismol (as directed by instruction label).
- Hydrate.
- Cold water.

SYMPTOMS: TRAUMA (BLUNT OR PENETRATING)

- Mild pain.
- Nausea.
- Pain worsened by flexing abdominal wall muscles.

⚠ **Red Flags:** Any hole in the skin or protruding bowel, pain that is progressively becoming more severe, pain worsened with any movement or palpation, pain in the shoulders after abdominal injury, bloating or persistent vomiting, fever, or any dizziness, rapid breathing, rapid pulse, or altered level of responsiveness. Evacuate any penetrating abdominal trauma.

Treatment

- Sips of cold water.
- Tylenol for pain.
- Protruding bowel covered with clean moist (sterile) gauze, with several dry layers of gauze affixed on top..
- Leave penetrating object in place and stabilized (*see* Wound Care).
- Have a low threshold for immediate evacuation with significant blunt abdominal trauma.

🚁 **Evacuate:** Any patient with abdominal pain who also has:

- Abdominal pain worsened with movement.

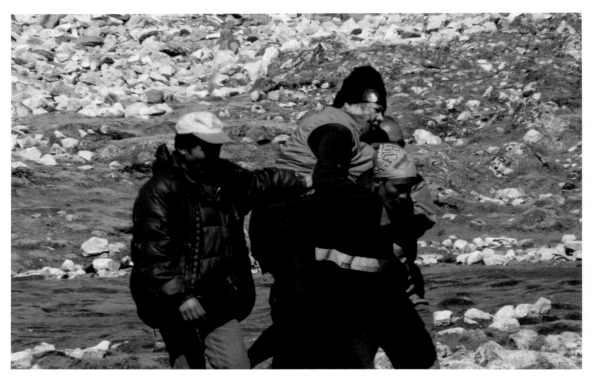

Sometimes abdominal pain can be a sign that surgical intervention is necessary. In this case, it is important to evacuate the patient. *Credit: Grant Lipman*

- Persistent localized pain for more than twelve hours.
- Intermittent diffuse pain lasting more than twenty-four hours.
- Black tarry stools.
- Fevers for eight hours with abdominal pain.
- Blood in vomit, stool, or urine (other than flecks of blood).
- Positive pregnancy test with abdominal pain.
- Inability to tolerate fluids.
- Combination of: sunken eyes, dry lining of the mouth, decreased urine output, and/or generalized weakness, dizziness.
- Any penetrating trauma.
- Blunt trauma with red flags.

3

ALLERGIC REACTION AND ANAPHYLAXIS

An allergic reaction can be set off by a bug bite, contact with a plant, or a food allergy. Symptoms of an allergic reaction range from mild to severe, the most severe of which is a life-threatening emergency called anaphylaxis. Most anaphylaxis will occur within one hour of onset of symptoms. People who develop anaphylaxis usually present with an allergic reaction initially that progresses. However, anaphylaxis can present abruptly as an isolated and catastrophic event. Allergic reactions can reoccur (rebound), so it is imperative to continue the entire course of treatment. Any patient who is suspected of having or is being treated for anaphylaxis should be immediately evacuated. Epinephrine is reserved for cases of severe allergic reaction and/or anaphylaxis; this is a potent prescription drug that can be

Insect bites or stings can cause allergic reactions.

dangerous to both provider and recipient if used incorrectly. Administrators need to be trained in the unique delivery of the drug.

SYMPTOMS

- **Mild (may be diffuse):** Red or blotchy skin, raised welts, itching, burning, red or watery eyes.
- **Moderate:** Skin rash and swelling to face or over entire body, sense of throat scratchiness or fullness, abdominal pain.
- **Severe/Anaphylaxis:** Shortness of breath, wheezing when breathing, tongue/lip swelling, inability to speak or only few word sentences, difficulty swallowing, and/or altered level of responsiveness.

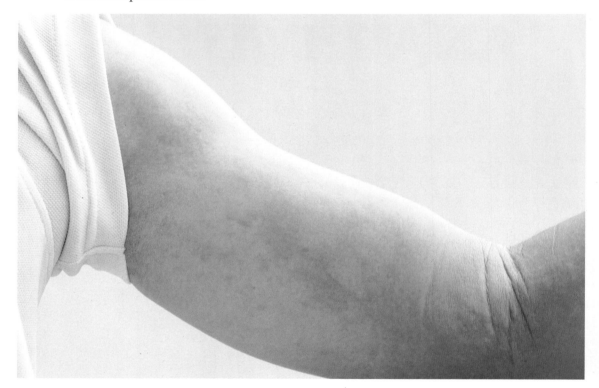

Blotchy, red skin or a rash is a sign of an allergic reaction.

⚠ **Red Flags:** Any symptom of moderate or severe allergic reaction or anaphylaxis.

Treatment

- Remove the offending allergen from the patient or the patient from the perceived offending trigger or environment.
- If a localized reaction, apply corticosteroid cream.
- **Mild and Moderate:** Benadryl and Pepcid (as directed by instruction label) for three days.
- **Severe/Anaphylaxis: <u>EpiPen instructions</u>:** 1) Pull off the safety cap. 2) Hold the EpiPen by grasping the shaft and placing the tip of the unit against the outer thigh, halfway between the hip and knee (ideally against the skin, but can be used through thin clothing). 3) Push the unit against the thigh until it clicks, which releases the hidden needle and delivery of medication. 4) Hold in place for a count of ten. May repeat in five to fifteen minutes if initial dose is ineffective or symptoms recur. Add all Mild and Moderate allergic reaction medicines.

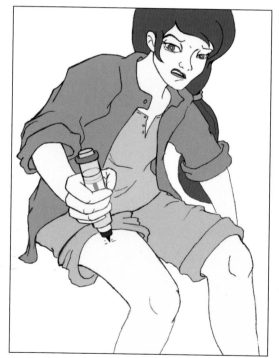

An EpiPen is an effective way to treat a severe allergic reaction or anaphylaxis.

Evacuate: Any patient who has received epinephrine. Any allergic reaction that does not improve with optimum treatment. Continue medications during evacuation.

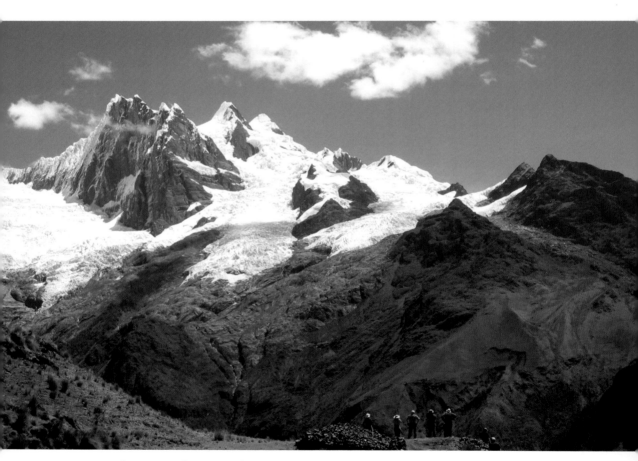

When traveling rapidly to altitudes above 8,000 feet, people are more likely to experience altitude illness. *Credit: Grant Lipman*

4

ALTITUDE ILLNESS

Altitude illness results from the body's inability to adjust to the relatively low ambient oxygen concentration in the atmosphere at high altitudes. The amount of oxygen in the air stays a relatively constant 21 percent, but as altitude is gained, the amount of oxygen in the air decreases with lowered barometric pressures. So there is less inhaled oxygen the higher one ascends. For example, at 19,000 feet (5,757 meters) there is half the barometric pressure as sea level, so about half the available oxygen per breath. The compensatory response of the body upon ascending to high altitude to optimize the delivery of oxygen to the tissues is called acclimatization. Acclimatization is best accomplished by a gradual graded ascent with rest days. For example, while someone in a hot air balloon who rapidly ascended to the height of Mount Everest (with 28 percent of the oxygen of sea level) would rapidly pass out and then die, people have successfully climbed the mountain without oxygen, because they acclimatized. A gradual ascent will maximize the chances for the body to successfully handle the stress of a relatively low oxygen environment, and allow one to feel well.

The body's normal response to high altitude includes an increased breathing rate to deliver the amount of oxygen to your body; increased urination; a fast heart rate; swelling of fingers, hands, and feet; and intermittent rapid breathing while sleeping, with brief breath holding spells. If someone is symptomatic with altitude illness (i.e., poorly acclimatized), descent to the last elevation where they felt well should resolve the symptoms. If someone is sick at high altitude, assume it is altitude sickness until proven otherwise.

Altitude illness usually affects people traveling above 6,500 to 8,000 feet (2,400 meters); it is a spectrum of disease ranging from mild to severe acute mountain sickness (AMS), high-altitude pulmonary edema (HAPE), or high-altitude cerebral edema (HACE). Mild to moderate AMS in the continental United States is most common. Remember that altitude illness may progress from an annoying headache, to debilitating sickness, to even fatal HACE. So early symptom recognition and evacuation to lower altitudes for moderate to severe disease may avoid a later rescue for a victim unable to walk or respond. There are many prescription medications for both prevention and treatment of altitude sickness.

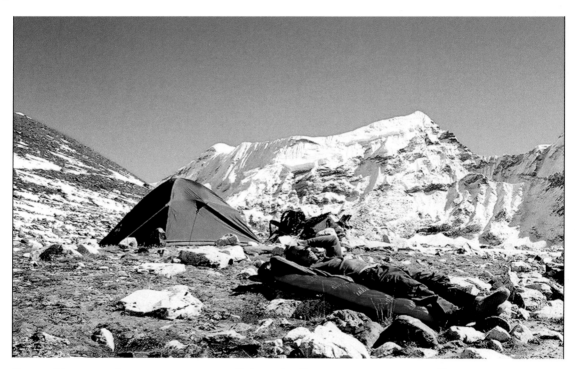

By paying attention to symptoms of altitude illness, a person can tell when they should stop ascending or descend to lower altitudes. A headache and fatigue may be early signs of acute mountain sickness. *Credit: Grant Lipman*

The most common prescription drug and considered the "gold standard" for both prevention and treatment of AMS is acetazolamide (Diamox). The drug is presumed to work by increasing the amount of urination, causing a compensatory increase in breathing and subsequent increase in the amount of delivered oxygen. The prevention dose is 125mg, twice per day; and the treatment dose for AMS is 250mg, twice per day. (Always follow the directions on the instruction label).

Acetazolamide is no substitute for safe ascent profiles, as many people get AMS while taking preventive doses of the drug if they go up too high too fast. If a person has mild to moderate symptoms of AMS, they can be treated with acetazolamide and stay at the altitude they are at. No one should be treated and continue to ascend until the AMS symptoms have resolved. If symptoms are severe or there is concern that evacuation may become difficult (from deteriorating weather or other reasons), it is best to descend to the last elevation the person felt well at. Once the AMS symptoms have resolved, the individual can ascend, taking the prevention dosage of acetazolamide if they are so inclined.

Ibuprofen is a common drug (600mg taken three times a day for one day, starting the morning of ascent) that has been shown to be very effective at preventing AMS. This drug has been rigorously studied at altitudes found in North America or Western Europe, and works well at these altitudes. Likely not as efficient as acetazolamide, but the ease of over-the-counter access and low side effect profile make it an attractive option. However, it should not be used for AMS prevention at elevations above 13,000 feet (4,000 meters), like those found in the mountains of Alaska, South America, or Asia.

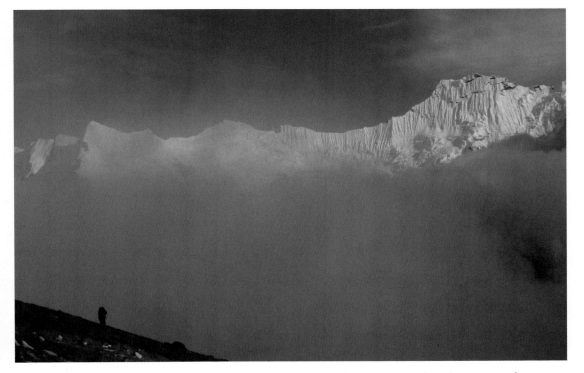

Ascending gradually gives your body time to naturally adjust to the decrease of oxygen per breath in the environment. *Credit: Grant Lipman*

Another prescription drug that is used for treatment of AMS and HACE is a steroid called dexamethasone. It is a powerful anti-inflammatory, and should never be used during ascent. Unlike acetazolamide, it does not assist with acclimatization, and may mask symptoms of altitude illness. So, if a person has taken dexamethasone (per the instruction label), it is prudent to stay at the altitude they are at for at least twenty-four hours to ensure they are asymptomatic before ascending (for moderate AMS), or to immediately descend (HACE and severe AMS).

High altitude cerebral edema presents as a severe form, or end stage, of AMS. There is progressive swelling in the brain that leads to severe headache and eventually altered level of responsiveness (LOR) that may present as confusion, amnesia, drowsiness, or unconsciousness. Another hallmark of the disease is ataxia, a gait imbalance that may present as inability to walk a straight line or loss of balance. HACE may arise as a progression of AMS symptoms, or in fulminant cases, present as a rapid neurologic deterioration without preceding symptoms of AMS. Dexamethasone and acetazolamide should be given, along with immediate descent. The person suffering for HACE should not be allowed to re-ascend, and as they are altered and unsteady, do not let them descend alone.

High altitude pulmonary edema is a disorder which presents with severe shortness of breath arising from an accumulation of excess fluid in the lung tissues and gas exchange spaces. Symptoms usually begin two to three days after ascent to high altitude, with progressive shortness of breath, cough, weakness on minimal exertion and fatigue. With greater accumulation of fluid there is severe shortness of breath, rapid heart rate, and a progressive cough that can become frothy or bloody with crackling or wheezing sounds. The person with HAPE needs to be recognized early, and descended to the last elevation they felt well at. Minimizing the amount of exertion will decrease the symptoms, so rest, backpack removal, or being carried (and oxygen if available) is ideal. Do not let this person descend alone. A decrease in as little as one thousand feet (three hundred meters) can lead to an improvement of symptoms. Once asymptomatic, the HAPE patient can (cautiously) re-ascend.

GUIDELINES FOR SAFE TRAVEL AT HIGH ALTITUDE:

- Ascend gradually to allow time for your body to naturally compensate to the physiologic stress of a lower oxygen environment.
- When traveling above 10,000 feet (3,300 meters), do not increase sleeping altitude by more than 1,650 feet (500 meters) each night.
- For every 3,300 feet (1,000 meters) gained in sleeping elevation, take a rest day.

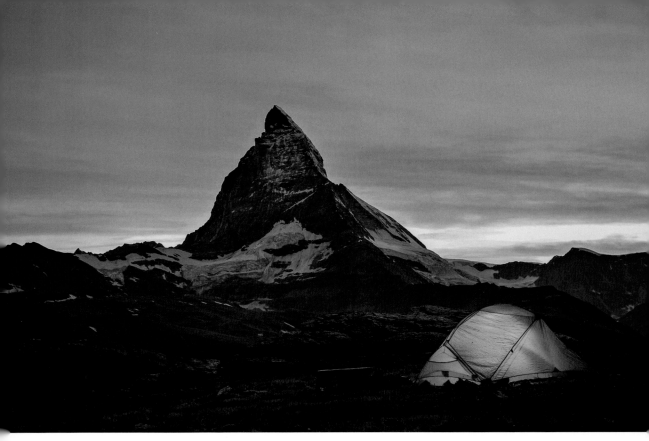

Don't increase sleeping altitude more than 1,650 feet each night when traveling at altitudes higher than 10,000 feet.

- If you feel sick at high altitude, assume it is altitude illness until proven otherwise.
- If you have mild symptoms at high altitude, do not ascend to a new sleeping altitude until you feel better.
- If you feel sick (mild symptoms) and are unable to feel normal (acclimatize) after twenty-four to thirty-six hours, descend to the last elevation where you felt well.
- If you feel sick (moderate to severe symptoms) at high altitude, descend to the last elevation where you felt well.
- Altitude illness is often more severe the morning after ascent. This should be taken into account when considering evacuation decisions in the afternoon or evening.

SYMPTOMS

- **Mild AMS:** Headache, nausea or vomiting, fatigue, poor sleep, lack of appetite, dizziness—similar to an alcoholic hangover.

- **Moderate/Severe AMS:** More severe or pronounced symptoms of AMS that may be debilitating. The patient is too fatigued and dizzy to walk any distances; vomiting and horrible headaches will occur.
- **HAPE:** Shortness of breath and/or rapid heart rate at rest or with mild exertion.
  - ➤ Dry cough, worse when lying flat (early in disease).
  - ➤ Wet cough, weakness, difficulty catching breath (later in disease).
  - ➤ Often begins on the second day after ascent to high altitude.

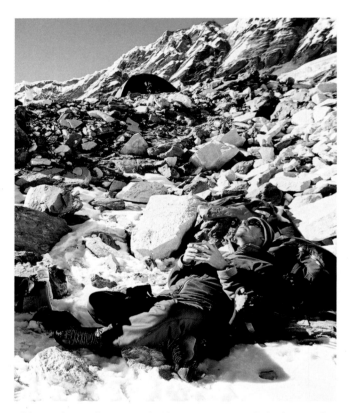

Severe shortness of breath and a cough that's worse while lying flat may be an early sign of high altitude pulmonary edema. *Credit: Grant Lipman*

- **HACE:** Altered level of responsiveness (LOR), inappropriate behavior, seizures, lethargy, or unconsciousness.
- Gait (walking) imbalance, loss of coordination.
- Severe headache.

⚠ **Red Flags:** Severe "ice pick" or "throbbing" headache on ascent, vomiting, any altered level of responsiveness, persistent elevated heart rate or breathing rate at rest.

Treatment

- **Mild AMS:** Maintain adequate hydration and nutrition.
  - ➤ Ibuprofen for headache (as directed by instruction label).
  - ➤ Do not ascend while feeling unwell.
  - ➤ Do not begin ascending until symptoms have completely resolved.
  - ➤ If symptoms do not improve in twenty-four to thirty-six+ hours, descend to last elevation where you felt well.
- **Moderate/Severe AMS:** Same as for mild AMS.
  - ➤ Immediate descent (at least one thousand feet or until patient feels better).
  - ➤ If possible, do not wait until morning for descent.

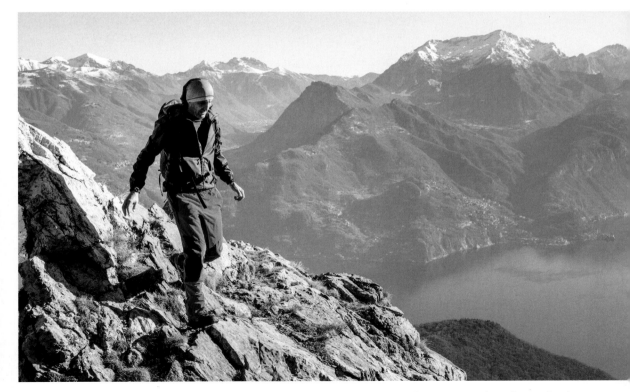

If moderate or severe altitude sickness hits you, begin descending immediately to the last elevation you felt well at.

- **HAPE/HACE:** Immediate descent (at least one thousand feet or until patient feels better).
  - ➢ If possible and safe to descend, do not wait until morning, as symptoms will likely worsen overnight, and the patient may not be able to walk out on his or her own power.

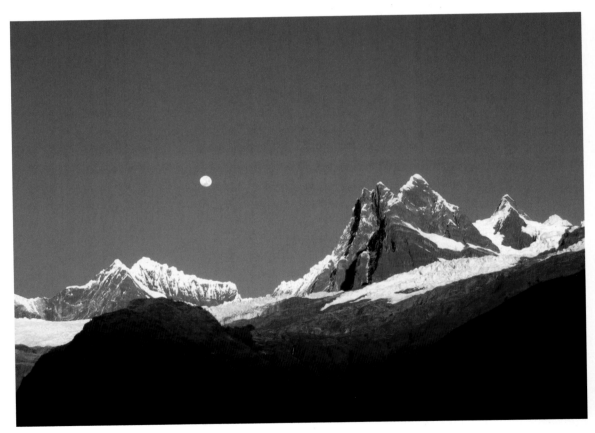 **Evacuate:**
- Any person who has HACE or HAPE.
- Any person with severe AMS that is not improving.
- Never allow a sick person to descend alone.

Credit: Grant Lipman

5

BLISTERS

Blisters are the most commonly reported injuries in the wilderness. While preventable and easily treatable, blisters can mean the difference between an enjoyable trip and incredible discomfort.

Preparation begins with properly fitting footwear. Size the boots in the evening (when the foot is most swollen), and break them in before a trip to accustom both boots and feet to ensure comfort. Cotton socks should be avoided; a synthetic sock or a combination of thin synthetic inner sock and thicker cushioning outer sock has been shown to minimize blister occurrence. Soft and supple feet are better able to withstand the sheer stress that causes blisters than hard and cracked feet. Feet should be kept well hydrated with lotion to keep them supple, and calluses should be filed down, and toe nails kept well trimmed.

A blisters starts with a hot spot, a sensation of heat that is a warning sign that needs to be recognized and immediately treated to avoid progression to a painful blister. Treating a blister as soon as possible improves outcome and reduces potential complications. The pain of a blister arises from pressure on the incompressible blister fluid between skin layers. Small blisters that do not cause discomfort should be left intact. Otherwise, blister fluid should be drained to minimize discomfort and to keep the protective roof of the blister intact. The drainage and treatment of blisters is done in a way to minimize the possibility of infection. Blood-filled blisters represent a deeper injury, and *should not* be drained. Likewise, blisters

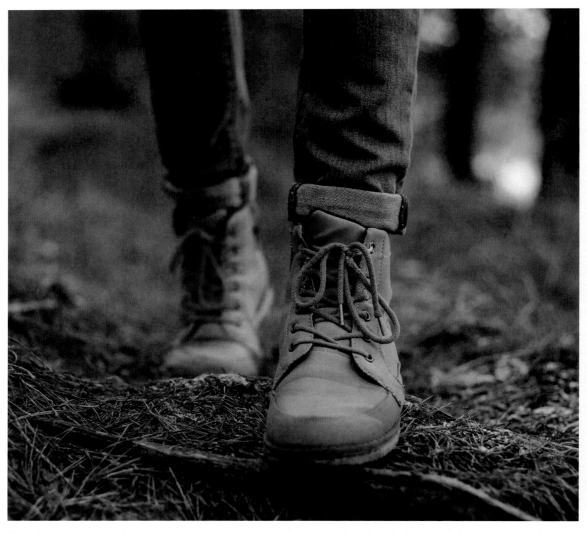

Break in boots before going on a trip to make sure that both feet will be comfortable.

underneath calluses should not be drained, as they are painful to access, may become infected, and re-accumulate fluid quickly. Keeping feet clean and dry (avoiding prolonged wetness) will lead to a lower incidence of blisters.

SYMPTOMS: HOT SPOT
- Warmth, rubbing, discomfort, pain, or raised or red area. No fluid accumulation.

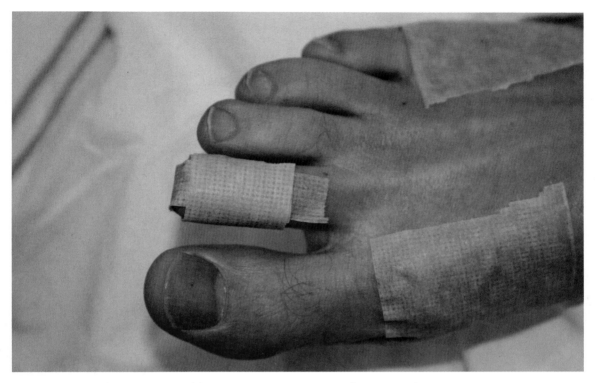

Hot spots can be prevented by pre-taping commonly irritated areas prior to starting an activity. *Credit: Grant Lipman*

Treatment

- Place a strip of paper tape over the hot spot. The length should overlap the healthy skin on either side by at least the width of the hot spot. Take care to ensure there are no "dog ears" or wrinkles, which may worsen the friction.

- **Prevention:** Apply paper tape to commonly irritated areas—pre-taping before starting your activity to prevent hot spots has been proven to be effective in preventing them.

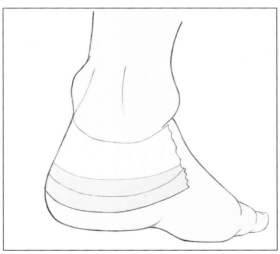

Paper tape–covered hot spot.

SYMPTOMS: BLISTER

- Fluid-filled bubble of skin. Painful.
- ⚠ **Red Flags:** Blood-filled blister, redness/streaking around blister, blisters beneath a callus.

Treatment

- Prepare both the blister skin and safety pin with an alcohol pad (the diameter of the safety pin is larger than a sewing needle to allow continuous drainage, yet not too large as to risk de-roofing the blister).
- Puncture blister with pin at several points on the blister wall (toward the outside of the foot), rather than one large hole. This will allow natural foot pressure to continually squeeze out fluid. One large hole may destroy the integrity of the blister's roof.
- Gently push fluid out with your fingers or gauze.
- Blot expressed fluid.
- Cover with paper tape (protects the blister roof when removed), overlapping blister by double its diameter on either side.
- Can cover with benzoin (for adhesion), then shaped adhesive tape (such as Elastikon) overlapping the paper tape (twice the diameter of the blister). Trim tape with rounded corners to minimize dog-ears and rolling off.
- Re-accumulated fluid can be drained through intact bandage.

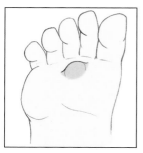 Blister.

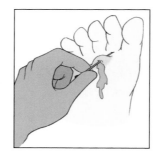 Draining a blister.

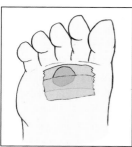 Paper tape covering a drained blister.

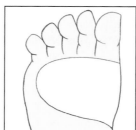 Elastikon tape covering a drained blister.

SYMPTOMS: OPEN/TORN BLISTER

Treatment

- Using small scissors, carefully unroof the blister (painless), completely trimming off the dead skin.
- Place Spenko 2nd Skin to cover the raw area.
- Cover with paper tape.
- Can cover with benzoin (for adhesion), then shaped adhesive tape (such as Elastikon) overlapping the paper tape (twice the diameter of the blister).
- Trim tape with rounded corners to minimize dog-ears and rolling off (as discussed with regular blisters).

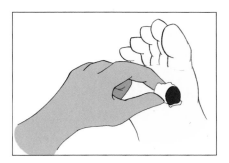

Unroofing a torn blister.

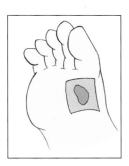

Spenko 2nd Skin–covered open blister.

SYMPTOMS: HEEL BLISTER

Treatment

- Treat open or closed blister as described in the steps above.
- Shape the "heel cup" by taking a length of Elastikon (or other adhesive) tape, cutting two midline incisions from either end, almost meeting in the middle, leaving a middle piece of tape intact. Looks like an *H* on its side.
- Trim all the corners.
- Apply benzoin for optimum adhesion.
- Apply the upper strip of the heel cup horizontally over the blister and intact skin above it.
- Wrap the lower two "wings" of the heel cup from under the heel up and perpendicular to the blister, with tension anchoring the wrap.
- Round off any corners or dog-ears with scissors.

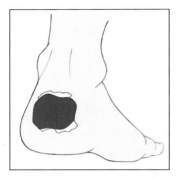

Heel blister.

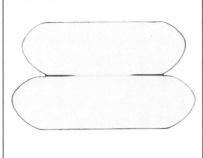

Elastikon tape cut for a heel cup.

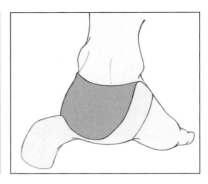

Wrapping the "wings" of a heel cup.

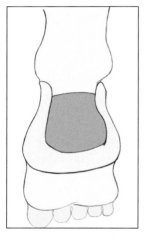

Completed heel cup.

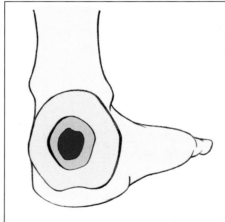

(Left) Moleskin "donut." Moleskin or Molefoam can be used on heel blisters to augment protection from a large blister. Cut a hole in the center slightly larger than the size of the blister, forming a donut shape, and place over the blister. Continue with all the steps of the above blister treatment.

SYMPTOMS: TOE BLISTERS

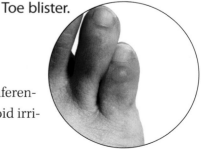

Toe blister.

Treatment

- Drain blister with prepared safety pin.
- Use one piece of paper tape to encircle the toe circumferentially (leaving tape end on top or bottom of toe to avoid irritating neighboring toes).
- Pinch closed.
- Trim sharp edges or wrinkles.
- Avoid cloth tape or Elastikon on toes, as abrasive tape will affect neighboring toes.

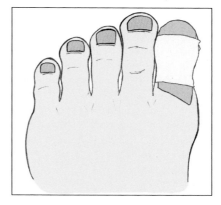

🚁 **Evacuate:** Few blister injuries require evacuation unless they are so painful that the person can't walk, or there are signs of an aggressive, spreading infection (pain with redness, streaking, pus from wound and/or fever).

SYMPTOMS: BLISTER UNDER TOENAIL (SUBUNGUAL HEMATOMA)

- Swollen, painful toe nail, with fluctuance at nail base.

Toe blister wrapped with paper tape. Note that toe pre-taping or hot spots can be wrapped the same way.

Treatment

- Take an 18-gauge hypodermic needle held perpendicular to the nail area of greatest fluctuance.
- Rotate back and forth between thumb and first finger, applying downward pressure.
- Continue until blood oozes freely.
- If painful, stop.
- Put pressure on nail to squeeze out excess fluid.
- Recap needle; can reuse, as these tend to recur.
- Wrap with paper tape like a toe blister.

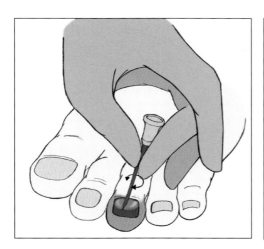

How to drain a subungual hematoma.

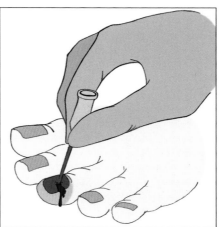

Draining a subungual hematoma.

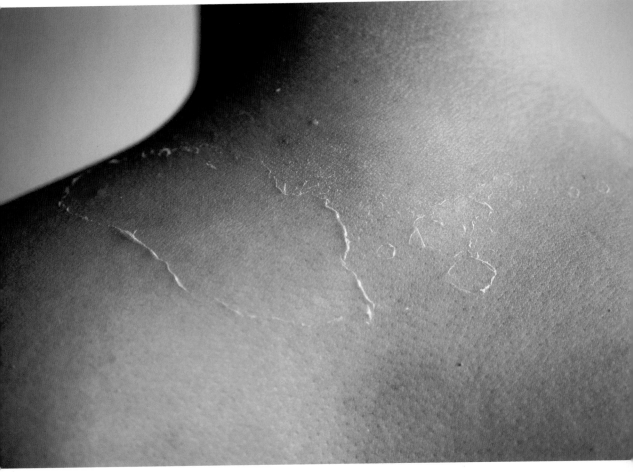

Sunburns are the most common kind of burn encountered in the wilderness.

6
BURNS

The most common burn in the wilderness is sunburn. Sunburn can be avoided by wearing hats and protective clothing, and by using high SPF sunblock with frequent reapplication. Both water and snow are surfaces which refract light and can worsen sunburns. Be especially cautious at high altitude, as ultraviolet light is increased by 4 percent to 6 percent every thousand feet (three hundred meters) in elevation.

Even small burns can be painful and debilitating and larger burns may predispose the victim to dehydration. Rapid cooling of the burnt area will minimize the amount of tissue damage, but avoid ice which can cause frostbite and damage the skin more. Burns can be divided into three categories depending on the extent or severity of the burn. *First-degree burns* involve the most superficial layer of the skin. It may be painful, but there are no blisters. If there is a large area of first-degree burn the victim may feel feverish and weak. *Second-degree burns* involve the next deeper layer of skin, with blister formation and more severe pain. *Third-degree burns* involve the full thickness of the skin and may be painless as nerves have been charred. There are no blisters and the skin may be white or hard. Third-degree burns will likely be ringed by second-degree burns, which are extremely painful. First-

Avoid sunburns with high SPF sunblock.

and second-degree burns are called *partial thickness burns,* and third-degree is a *full thickness burn* that usually requires a skin graft for healing.

Like all wounds in the backcountry, burns have the potential to become infected. Large burns should be considered for early evacuation for wound care, prevention of infection, and dehydration. Blisters can be left intact if they are not at risk for spontaneous rupturing. If large and fluctuant or possibly infected (turbid and filled with milky fluid), they should be carefully drained (*see* **Blisters**). Evaluate the lungs and breathing for any difficulties breathing that may represent a burn to the airway. Measure the size of a burn with your hand (palm of hand = approximately 1 percent of total body surface area), or per body surface area involved.

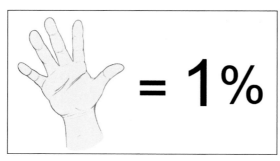

(Left) Estimation of the burn size with the palm of hand.

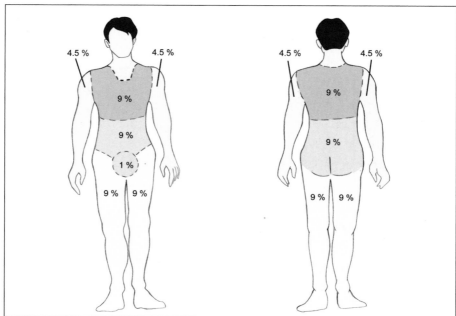

Estimation of the burn size by body surface area.

SYMPTOMS

- **Superficial:** Reddened skin and pain (similar to a sunburn).
- **Partial Thickness:** Red skin and blistered, skin may be pale white/yellow, severe pain.
- **Full Thickness:** Flesh may be charred, no pain (nerve endings are burned).

⚠️ **Red Flags:** Burns involving the face, mouth, airway, neck, hands, feet, or genitals.

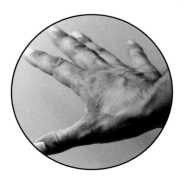

First-degree burn.

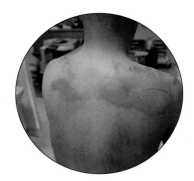

Second-degree burn.

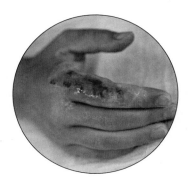

Third-degree burn.

Treatment

- Ensure the scene is safe.
- Extinguish burning clothes or material.
- Remove constricting clothes/jewelry.
- Immediately soak or copiously flush the burn with cool water (ideally for fifteen to twenty minutes).
- Wash burns with soap and drinkable water.
- Dress burn with antibiotic ointment (such as Polysporin) and nonstick gauze.
- Cover blisters with gauze dressing.
- Elevate involved extremity (to minimize swelling).
- Motrin or Tylenol for pain, per the instruction label.
- Aggressive hydration.
- Monitor for infection (change bandage every day, observe for redness/streaking/pus from wound).

🚁 **Evacuate:**

- Partial thickness burns involving more than 10 percent body surface area.
- Any full thickness burn.

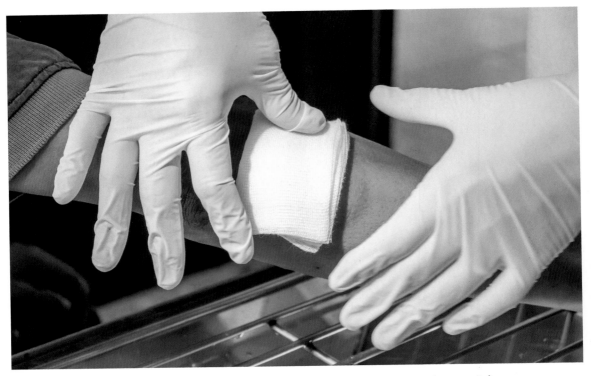

After washing the burns, dress them with antibiotic ointment and nonstick gauze.

- Any burn to the mouth, face, neck, genitals, and/or full circumference of any extremity: fingers, hands, or feet.
- Any burn that may have involved the airway (smoke inhalation), patient with cough, wheeze, singed nasal hair, or soot in nose or mouth.

7

CARDIOPULMONARY RESUSCITATION (CPR)

To check for unresponsiveness and establish the need for CPR, attempt to make verbal contact in a clear and loud voice. If unsuccessful, touch the shoulder gently and repeat. If there is a need to perform CPR on someone who is not breathing, the American Heart Association recommends initiating chest compressions without checking for pulses. Open the airway using the head-tilt/chin-lift procedure to ensure the tongue is not blocking the airway (*see* **Primary Assessment).** If there is no spontaneous breathing and the victim is unconscious, begin chest compressions.

The standards for performing CPR are well established by the American Heart Association. While CPR can be an effective life-sustaining intervention in the short term, the victim's survival rate after more than twenty minutes of CPR is very low. While CPR should be initiated when indicated,

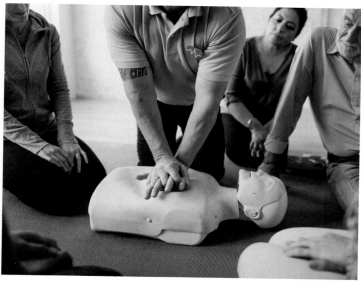

CPR classes allow you to practice proper technique with a mannequin.

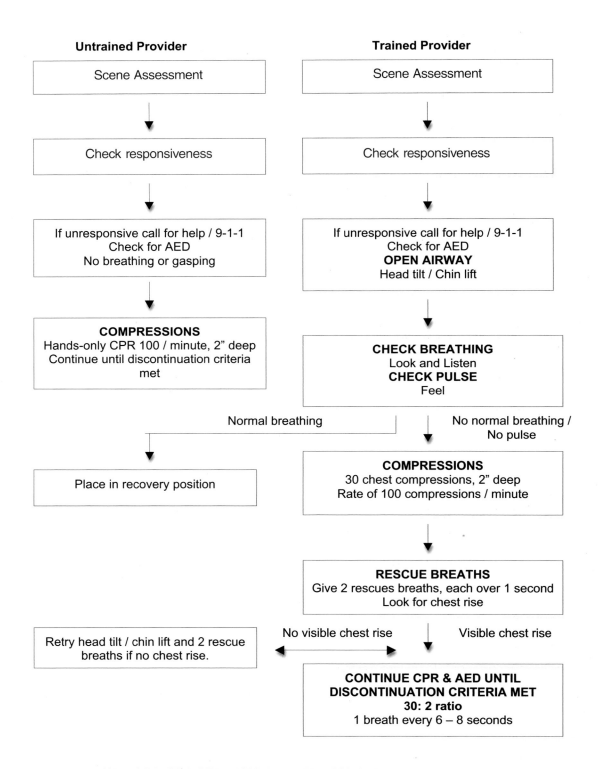

Untrained Provider

Scene Assessment

↓

Check responsiveness

↓

If unresponsive call for help / 9-1-1
Check for AED
No breathing or gasping

↓

COMPRESSIONS
Hands-only CPR 100 / minute, 2" deep
Continue until discontinuation criteria
met

Trained Provider

Scene Assessment

↓

Check responsiveness

↓

If unresponsive call for help / 9-1-1
Check for AED
OPEN AIRWAY
Head tilt / Chin lift

↓

CHECK BREATHING
Look and Listen
CHECK PULSE
Feel

Normal breathing ←

↓ No normal breathing /
No pulse

Place in recovery position

COMPRESSIONS
30 chest compressions, 2" deep
Rate of 100 compressions / minute

↓

RESCUE BREATHS
Give 2 rescues breaths, each over 1 second
Look for chest rise

No visible chest rise ← → Visible chest rise

Retry head tilt / chin lift and 2 rescue
breaths if no chest rise.

**CONTINUE CPR & AED UNTIL
DISCONTINUATION CRITERIA MET**
30: 2 ratio
1 breath every 6 – 8 seconds

early alerting of EMS for definitive care if possible is of utmost importance. These CPR protocols are not intended to be comprehensive and are no substitute for taking a CPR class, and every wilderness first responder should consider getting certified in CPR. While there are some exceptions to the rule in lightning, drowning, and hypothermia, CPR in the wilderness is rarely successful.

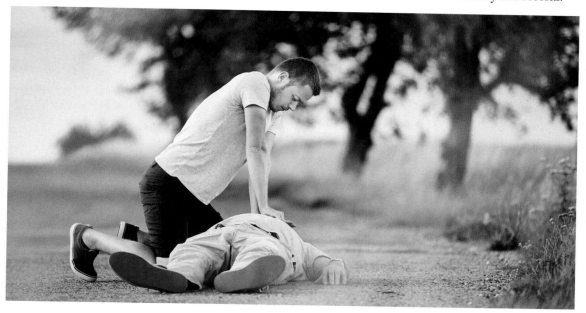

Train in CPR before going into the wilderness—you'll never know when you'll need the training.

CONTRAINDICATIONS TO CPR IN THE WILDERNESS

- Do not initiate CPR if there is:
  - ➤ Patient responsiveness.
  - ➤ Danger to rescuers, such that initiating CPR would put the rescuers at risk of harm.
  - ➤ Obvious lethal injury (i.e., decapitation).
  - ➤ A well-defined "Do Not Resuscitate (DNR)" status.

DISCONTINUATION OF CPR IN THE WILDERNESS

Once initiated, CPR should be continued until (any one of the following):

- Patient is responsive.
- The rescuers are exhausted.

- The rescuers are placed in danger.
- Patient care is turned over to EMS for definitive care.

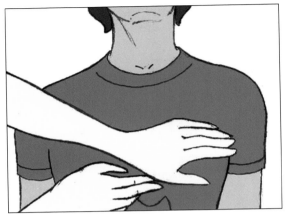

Hand position on the body for CPR.

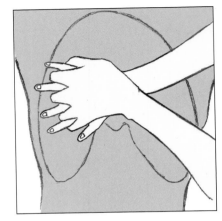

Hand position for CPR.

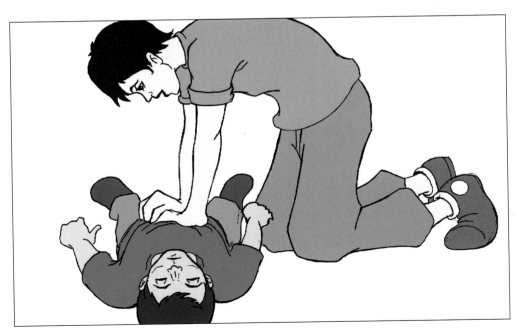

Body position for CPR.

8
CHEST PAIN

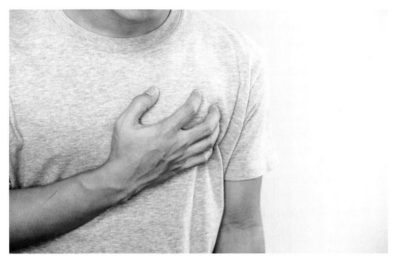

Do not ignore persistent chest pain; it could be a sign of a major issue.

Differentiating the causes of chest pain or chest pressure is challenging in the wilderness. Chest pain can be a benign infection from a viral irritant, which is often a sharp pain and reproducible when pushing on the chest wall. It may be a more serious (and potentially fatal) problem in the lungs like a blood clot (pulmonary embolism). Women on birth control are especially at risk for this, which may present gradually or suddenly, with sharp chest pain, worse on inspiration with shortness of breath—often exacerbated by lying down or exertion. Ask the patient if there is a history of heart disease or blood clots (or family history of this), or if they are currently taking medicine for high blood pressure. If so, assist them with taking the prescribed medications. Younger people may complain of persistent rapid heart rate rather than pain. While it is better to avoid exerting a patient with concerning chest symptoms, it may be timelier and more advantageous to have them ambulate to assist in the evacuation. If a patient has persistent chest pain, consider not moving the patient and bringing medical care to them.

A heart attack may present with the following symptoms: chest pain, heaviness, or shortness of breath that is exacerbated with exertion. Radiation of pain to the neck, left arm, or back, possibly with sweating and clammy skin. This is due to an inadequate supply of oxygenated blood to the heart muscle from an obstructed or narrowed blood vessel (artery) in the heart. The chest pain may be stress on the heart (ischemia) or cell death (infarction). This is difficult to differentiate in the wilderness, so assume the worst case scenario. Allowing the person to rest will minimize the stress on heart, and exerting them further will exacerbate the heart's oxygen demand and may lead to further damage to the heart muscle. Death from a heart attack is usually caused by an irregular heart beat that cannot sustain life, or a weakened muscle that cannot adequately pump blood. Early symptom recognition and prompt evacuation will hopefully minimize the chances for a bad outcome.

In some rare cases the large vessel (aorta) leading from your heart can have a tear in it. This is an aortic dissection, and is more common in people with a history of high blood pressure. The classic symptoms are a tearing intense pain, with a rapid onset and peak that radiates into the chest. While this may be challenging to differentiate from a heart attack, it requires prompt evaluation by a doctor and evacuation to definitive medical care.

Sometimes a person's heart can beat in a very rapid rate that may be in a regular or irregular rhythm. This rapid heart rate (tachycardia) may occur due to heat illness, exertion, high altitude, trauma, or pain. If the tachycardia occurs suddenly without exacerbating events, it is likely primarily a heart problem. The symptoms include a feeling of rapid heart beating ("palpitations"), skipping beats, chest tightness, lightheadedness, or weakness. There are several maneuvers to slow down the rapid heart rate without medications, These include: taking a deep breath and while pursing one's lips, bear down hard; taking a deep breath and plunging a face into cold water; or pressing gently but firmly on closed eyelids for fifteen to twenty seconds. If unable to break this cycle, it may necessitate an evacuation.

In some cases the heart beats too slow (bradycardia), and the decreased amount of oxygenated blood to the brain can cause dizziness or even a loss of consciousness. This is usually in response to a painful event, rapid change in position, or emotional stimulus. Bradycardias are rarely a primary heart malfunction, and if due to the heart muscle malfunction, hypothermia, or rare international disease in conjunction with an elevated temperature, patient should be rapidly evacuated for further care and evaluation.

SYMPTOMS

- Chest pain, tightness, or pressure.
- Pain radiating to the left arm or jaw.
- Weakness, nausea, shortness of breath, pale skin, and/or sweating with the pain.
- Lightheaded or dizzy.

⚠ **Red Flags:** Chest pressure that is worsened by activity, reduced by resting and/or associated with sweating. Sharp, sudden onset of chest pain with difficulty breathing.

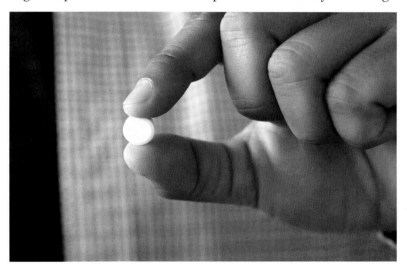

If the patient has their own medication, have them take it. Aspirin is another treatment option.

Treatment

- Reduce activity and anxiety. Place patient in a position of comfort.
- If patient has nitroglycerin, have him take his own medicine as directed.
- Give aspirin as directed by the instruction label.
- If symptoms occur at high altitude (10,000 feet plus), reduce altitude by at least 1,000 feet (300 meters).
- For younger patients with rapid heart rate, have them forcibly "hum" for thirty to sixty seconds, which can increase the firing of nerves and thus slow down the heart rate.

🚁 **Evacuate:**

- Any patient with chest pain worsened by exertion or persistent chest pain (twenty minutes or more).

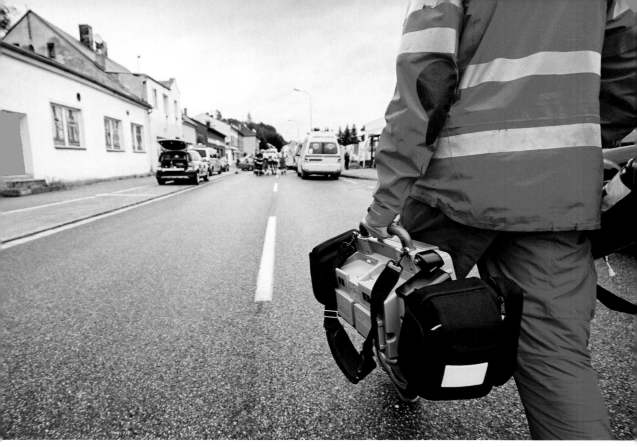

If the patient's chest pain increases with movement, try to bring EMS to them.

- Patient with persistent rapid pulse (one hundred beats per minute or more) or with associated shortness of breath and/or chest pain.
- If pain or shortness of breath is worsened by exertion, it may be of benefit to bring EMS to the patient, rather than have the patient walk out in distress.

9

CHEST TRAUMA

With trauma to the chest wall, force can break or bruise ribs, collapse the underlying lung, or cause bruising and bleeding in the lung. Even bruised ribs can be very painful with usually an increased amount of pain on deep inhalation. While injured ribs may make movement and exertion painful, the life-threatening concerns are injury to the underlying lung and blood vessels. A collapsed lung (pneumothorax) is caused by a leak of air into the potential space between the lung tissue and chest wall. As this air accumulates and expands, it exerts pressure on the lung which can then collapse with progressive pain, breathing difficulty, shortness of breath, and even collapse and death from pressure on the internal blood vessels (tension pneumothorax). Spontaneous pneumothorax can occur with a sudden complaint of difficulty breathing and/or sharp chest pain, worsened on deep breaths in the absence of trauma. A bruised

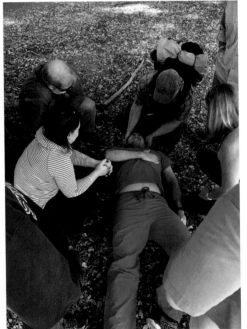

If the patient's chest is tender on touch or it is painful for them to take a deep breath, they may be experiencing chest trauma.

lung injury may have a delayed presentation of progressive shortness of breath and difficulty breathing after trauma, so careful observation is important for up to twelve hours after initial injury.

SYMPTOMS

- Reproducible chest wall or back tenderness on touching.
- Pain on taking a deep breath.
- Sensation of being unable to take a deep breath.

⚠ **Red Flags:** Severe shortness of breath, passing out, "rice crispy" sensation over injury site, bubbles or gushing air exiting from chest wound.

Treatment

- Place the patient in a position of comfort or on the non-injured side.
- For *reproducible* rib pain, wrap painful ribs with a circumferential compression bandage (like a girdle), effectively "buddy taping" the area like you would splint a broken finger.
- Ibuprofen and acetaminophen for pain, per the instruction labels.
- Encourage patient to periodically take deep breaths (to inflate the lungs).

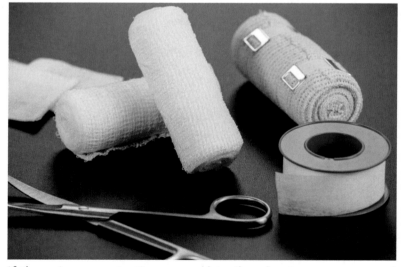

If there is a penetrating wound to the chest, use gauze and other supplies to seal the wound.

- If penetrating wound to chest with bubbles and/or air, affix sterile/clean gauze over wound, make an airtight seal by *taping on three sides* (leaving fourth side of bandage untaped to allow for air to exit and prevent air trapping in the lungs).

Evacuate:

- Any symptoms of difficulty breathing or shortness of breath after chest trauma.
- Any coughing up of blood after chest injury.
- Any air bubbles/gush of air from chest wound.
- Cough producing sputum and/or fever.
- Persistent severe pain that limits ability to take comfortable breaths or walk normally, despite appropriate pain medicine and buddy taping chest wall.

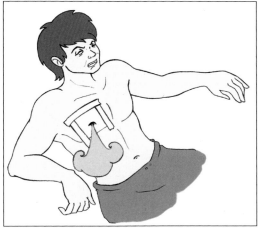

Chest trauma.

If the patient continues to cough up blood after a chest injury, you may need to evacuate.

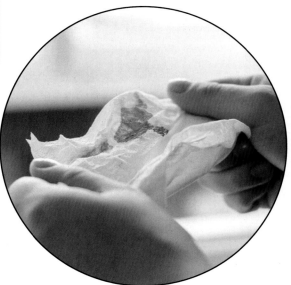

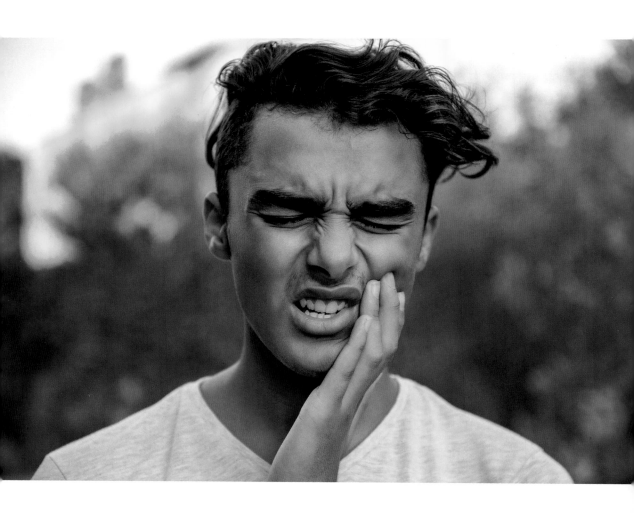

10

DENTAL PAIN

Dental pain can be remarkably severe, but while potentially debilitating from discomfort, it is rarely due to a reason that will necessitate an evacuation. Tooth pain occurs in areas that have eroded due to a cavity, a traumatic injury, or a lost filling, To localize the problem tooth, tap each one individually to find the point of tenderness. If there is swelling (inflammation) to the base of the tooth or the gum and surrounding structures, the pain may be more dispersed. If there is localized gum swelling with an obvious soft and fluctuant area, this is a collection of pus called an abscess, and the drainage of this (with a cleaned needle or tip of a blade where the gum meets the tooth) will relieve some of the pressure and pain. If a tooth has been dislodged from trauma, and is partially attached, do not attempt to remove it as it could damage the root of the tooth. Rather, leave it alone and evacuate to see a dentist as soon as possible for optimal dental results. Any tooth that has been fully dislodged should not be scrubbed (which can injure the root and inhibit reattachment). Rather, gently rinse and keep moist (either between the cheek and gum if no risk of being swallowed or in a waterproof container), and be evaluated by a dentist as soon as possible for best chance at reimplantation.

It's rare that dental pain will require an evacuation, but it does help to know how to treat it.

SYMPTOMS

- Extreme tooth sensitivity to hot or cold stimulus.
- Swelling of gum or cheek
- Visually or palpably identifiable tooth irregularity.

⚠ **Red Flags:** Severe swelling to gum or cheek with or without fever.

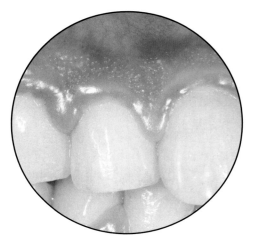

Swollen gums can be a sign of a larger problem, such as a bacterial infection.

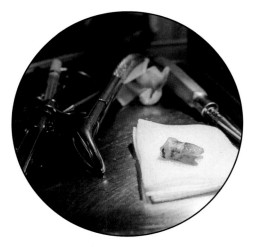

If a tooth is knocked out and cannot be replaced, do not scrub it, and wrap it in clean gauze so that a professional can replace it later.

Treatment

- If a crown or filling is lost or the tooth breaks, cover the edge or "hole" with soft candle wax or sugarless gum; bite down to get a good approximation.
- Ibuprofen and acetaminophen for pain, per the instruction labels.
- Avoid very hot or cold liquid or food. If the tooth is knocked out of the socket, irrigate the tooth with drinkable water and attempt to replace it in the socket. Do NOT scrub the roots to clean. Make a "splint" of neighboring teeth using cooled soft candle wax or dental floss tied around opposing teeth. If tooth cannot be replaced, wrap in sterile/clean gauze, and have patient carry the tooth between their cheek and gum if not at risk to be inhaled into the lungs.

🚁 **Evacuate:**

- Any patient with a tooth knocked out of the socket.
- Any broken tooth with severe pain.
- Increasing swelling to cheek or gum with or without fever.

11

DIABETIC EMERGENCIES

Diabetes is a disease where the body is unable to sufficiently break down sugar. Diabetes is usually well maintained and managed in a wilderness setting. There is often an increased caloric demand during wilderness activities from an increased amount of exercise, yet insulin dose requirements often drop. The diabetic should plan with their doctor prior to embarking on a wilderness adventure. Diabetic emergencies arise because there is a mismatch between the amount of sugar (glucose) in the blood and the body's ability to utilize that sugar (too much or too little insulin). Diabetics in a wilderness setting should consider checking their blood sugar with frequency, as well as familiarizing the trip leader or colleagues with personal testing apparatus, medicines, and ensuring their trip partners are able to identify signs and treatments of low blood sugar (hypoglycemia). The diabetic should plan

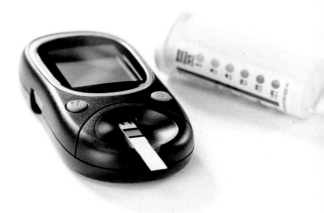

Diabetics should plan ahead and make sure to have supplies, such as a glucometer and medication, readily available.

ahead for optimum storage and administration of supplies (glucometer; spare batteries; duplicate medications such as insulin, pills, glucose paste; syringes; and ketone strips), and establish a sick day plan. Also plan to have routine meal times.

Insulin and cold: Avoid having insulin freeze. Keep next to skin in freezing temperatures, and if frozen solid, do not thaw and use.

Insulin and heat: Avoid prolonged direct sunlight and temperatures in excess of body temperature. Store wrapped within a sock next to a cool water bottle and/or in insulated case to retain coolness. Prolonged warmth may degrade efficacy of insulin, so test sugars more frequently.

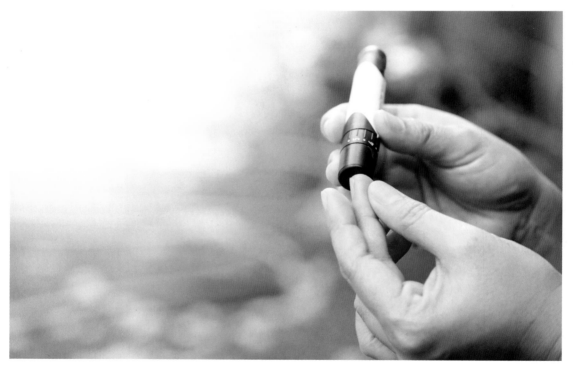

Insulin may be less efficient with prolonged heat or cold, so make sure to store insulin carefully, carry a backup supply, and to check sugar levels frequently.

Insulin should be administered by the patient only.

If unsure whether a diabetic who has an altered level of responsiveness (LOR) is suffering from too little sugar or too much, it is better to assume a low sugar state and to give sugar.

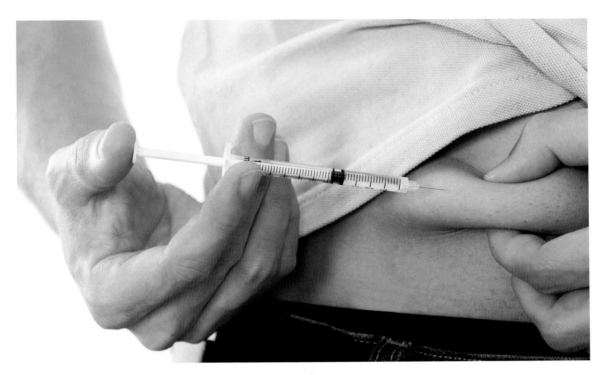

The patient should administer their own insulin.

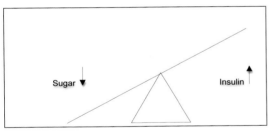

Hypoglycemia.

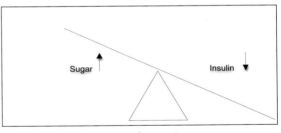

Hyperglycemia.

SYMPTOMS

- **Low blood sugar:** Rapid onset (minutes to hours).
  - ➢ Weak, sweating, confused, slurred speech, agitated, headache, seizure. They may appear drunk.
- **High blood sugar:** Slow onset (over a day).
  - ➢ Fatigue, hunger, excessive thirst, excessive urination, abdominal pain, nausea, vomiting, weakness, or blurred vision.
  - ➢ Possible preceding infectious symptoms.

⚠ **Red Flags:** Change in level of responsiveness, increasing thirst and/or urination.

Treatment

- Low Blood Sugar (under 60 mg/dL)
  - ➤ Check blood sugar using the patient's glucometer.
  - ➤ If conscious, give sugar/sugar water/candy, then complex carbohydrates such as a sandwich.
  - ➤ If unconscious, rub sugar/sugar containing gel on inside of cheek or under the tongue.
  - ➤ Once patient regains consciousness, give food to maintain normal blood sugar levels (80–120 mg/dL).

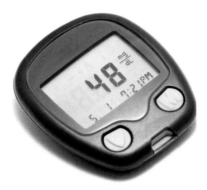

If a patient has low blood sugar, give them some sugar and carbohydrates so they can reach and maintain normal sugar levels.

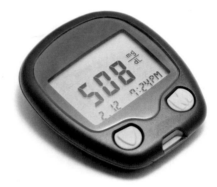

If they have very high blood sugar, then they need to hydrate and evacuate.

- High Blood Sugar (over 300 mg/dL)
  - ➤ Check blood sugar using the patient's glucometer.
  - ➤ Aggressive hydration and evacuation.

🚁 **Evacuate:**
- Any patient with diabetes who has lost consciousness or has prolonged changes in level of responsiveness for more than one hour.
- Persistent vomiting or diarrhea.
- Any diabetic patient who cannot (or will not) moderate his or her blood sugar levels.

12

DROWNING

Drowning is an event when the airways inhale (aspirate) water with subsequent breathing impairment. Drowning outcomes range from no disease, to some breathing difficulties and disease, to death. Terms to avoid are "submersion," "immersion," "near-drowning," "dry drowning," or "secondary drowning." If water is inhaled into the lungs, symptoms present quickly and progress; they do not suddenly appear days later. There is not a difference in salt-water versus fresh-water drowning, as it is the amount of water entering the lungs that produce symptoms. Always consider a traumatic injury (and possible spinal injury) in drowning victims if they have lost consciousness after diving into the water, as spinal precautions may be warranted.

In the event of a drowning resuscitation, do not attempt to push the water out through Heimlich or abdominal thrusts like you would a choking victim. Rather, approach the resuscitation like you would with anyone requiring CPR. However, in drowning the heart has usually stopped beating because of a lack of oxygen (asphyxia) in the lungs. Because this is typically a respiratory arrest that has caused a lack of a heart beat and pulse, rescue breathing should be started promptly, even while the victim is in shallow water. Resuscitations and CPR may have better outcomes in drowning than a primary cardiac (heart) event. There have been complete and successful resuscitations in cold water drownings due to hypothermia, so CPR should be continued for longer periods in such situations.

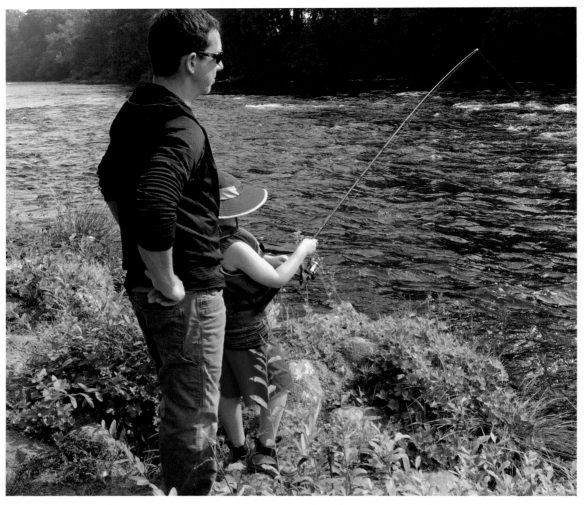

Make sure an adult is supervising any activities by the water. *Credit: Grant Lipman*

SAFETY AND PREVENTION

- All water-related activities should be supervised by a responsible adult.
- It only takes seconds to inhale small amounts of water and a child can drown in seconds when an adult is not looking.
- Utilize the "buddy system"—do not swim alone.
- Be aware of weather conditions; if strong winds or thunderstorms and lightning are in the area, get out of the water and seek shelter.

- Be aware of waves and rip currents. If you are caught in a rip current and being taken away from the beach, swim parallel to the shore until you are free from the current, then swim toward the shore.
- Everyone involved in a boating activity should wear a properly fit life jacket. A flotation toy is not an appropriate substitute.

SYMPTOMS

- Rapid breathing rate, shortness of breath, cough, wheezing, altered level of responsiveness (LOR), unconsciousness.

⚠ **Red Flags:** Any breathing difficulties, persistent coughing (more than five minutes).

Treatment

- Ensure scene safety for the rescuer.
- Get patient onto dry land.

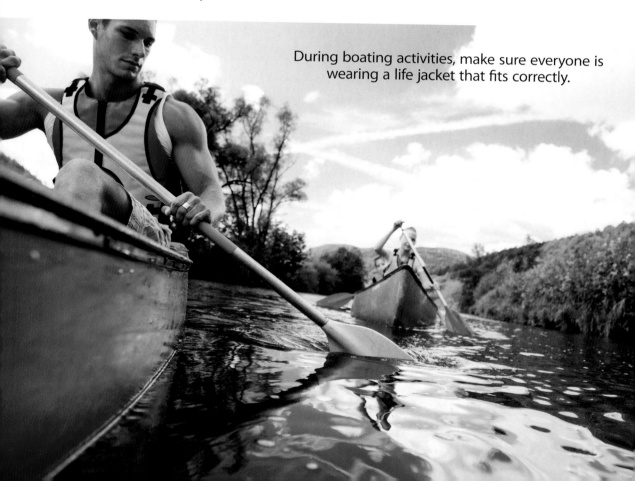

During boating activities, make sure everyone is wearing a life jacket that fits correctly.

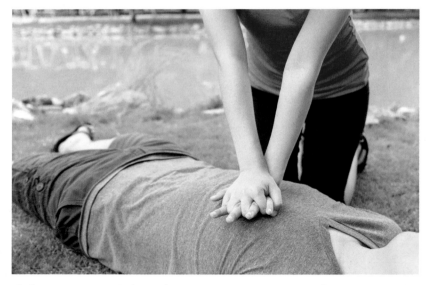

If the patient isn't breathing, initiate CPR once they are on dry land.

- Ensure spinal injury precautions if the victim was doing something that may have caused that (such as diving). (Refer to the FACS list given on page 283)
- Initiate aggressive CPR (rescue breaths and/or chest compressions) if not breathing and/or no pulse.
- Be mindful of wet clothing, and initiate hypothermia preventive care early.
- Observe for any symptoms of breathing difficulty.

Evacuate:
- Any patient who has lost consciousness.
- Any issues with breathing—persistent shortness of breath or cough, rapid breathing rate, "crackly" breathing sounds, blue discoloration around mouth—and/or altered level of responsiveness (LOR).

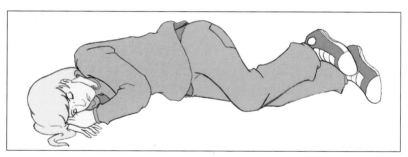

Recovery position.

13

EYES, EARS, NOSE, AND THROAT

Injuries and illnesses to the eyes can range from irritating to debilitating or even devastating. The most important thing with eyes is to note preceding trauma, symptom progression, and/or contact lens use. Contact lenses predispose people to more severe infections. Eye infections can be viral or bacterial and involve different depths of the eye structure. Progressive redness, a foreign body sensation, sensitivity to light, or change in visual acuity are all concerning symptoms that have limited management options in a wilderness environment, so symptoms such as these require evacuation for further care and evaluation. An infection or swelling to the eyelid (stye) should be treated with frequent (four times a day) warm compresses which can resolve it, or bring it to a head and allow it to self-drain. A foreign body lodged in the eye or underneath the eyelid is incredibly painful, but examination and eversion of the eyelid may be able to find an imbedded object, and gentle blotting may remove the offending substance. Bright and reflective surfaces such as snow, water, or sand can predispose to a sunburn to the cornea, the surface of the eye. This "snow blindness" is incredibly painful, and the pain and light sensitivity lead to a lack of vision due to inability to tolerate sunlight. Patching the eye, or cutting small slits in an eye covering, will limit the number of ultraviolet rays, decrease the pain, and make wilderness movement more negotiable. Ibuprofen for the pain is advised, and like any bad sunburn, it is self-limited and once endured is rarely repeated. Spontaneous loss of vision or visual field can be due to many reasons, from an injury to the light-receptive layers in the back of the eyeball to a problem with the blood vessels or nerves that feed the eye; regardless of the cause, loss of vision is a medical emergency that requires evacuation and emergent evaluation by an ophthalmologist.

Problems to the ears usually involve pain, trauma, change in hearing, or drainage. Ear pain (even with a fever) is usually an infection caused by a virus, which may resolve on its own without the need for antibiotics. Even a draining ear will usually resolve on its own. This is usually the same for facial/sinus pain and pressure, which is typically caused by viruses and managed by over-the-counter pain medicine.

Nose bleeds usually originate for injured blood vessels along the middle partition (septum) of the nose. Direct pressure is the best way to stop the bleed, but first the blood clot needs to be evacuated so it will not stent open the nostrils and inhibit the pressure point. After copiously blowing the nose, the victim will need to pinch the nostrils for ten to fifteen minutes. This is a long time to apply direct pressure, and it is more feasible to fashion a clothespin type apparatus by longitudinally cutting a green twig that can then be clamped over the nostrils. Nose bleeds are common in the mountains and can be due to irritation to the nasal lining by dry air. Preventive application of an antibiotic ointment or petroleum-based ointment to the nasal septum can lubricate the fragile mucosal lining and help minimize the fragile blood vessels.

Sore throats are most commonly caused by viruses. While uncomfortable, the pain, hoarse voice, swollen neck lymph nodes, and often fever is self-limited and treated with over-the-counter anti-inflammatories and salt-water gargles. In rare cases, the sore throat may represent a serious bacterial infection that may track to the deep tissues of the mouth and neck. This presents as severe pain, often with a high fever, difficulty opening the mouth, tenderness to the floor of the mouth or front of the neck, or a muffled "hot potato" voice. This needs to be evacuated.

SYMPTOMS: EYES

- Foreign body sensation, pain, irritation, tearing, redness, sensitivity to light.
- Severe pain/light sensitivity twelve hours after extended exposure to bright/reflected sunlight (possible snow blindness).
- Specks or "floaters" in vision.

⚠ **Red Flags:** Colored drainage from eyes, pain and redness in only one eye, loss of vision, or new "floaters."

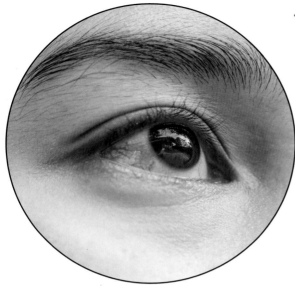

If you have blood or redness in one eye and it isn't painful, this is likely nothing to worry about. However, if you feel pain, it is a red flag.

Treatment

- If foreign body sensation, irrigate with drinkable water.
- If foreign body visualized, dab at it with moist clean cloth or cotton swab. Avoid scraping or rubbing the foreign body, as that may increase damage to the eye.
- If painless blood to white portion of eye, do nothing. This is not dangerous.
- If impaled object in eye, stabilize object with gauze padding and tape, and patch both eyes.
- If possible "snow blindness" (sunburn to the eyeball), patch eyes or keep covered. (If no sunglasses, consider using cloth or duct tape or a survival blanket with small slits or pinprick holes to see through). Ibuprofen and acetaminophen (as directed by the instruction label) for pain.

SYMPTOMS: EARS

- Ear pain, tenderness to manipulation of external ear, foreign body sensation, drainage from the ear.

Treatment

- Ear should be flushed with warm water via an irrigation syringe.
- Ibuprofen and acetaminophen for pain, per the instruction labels.

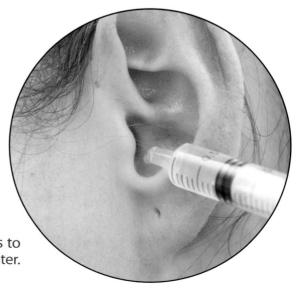

One way to treat ear pain is to flush it with warm water.

SYMPTOMS: NOSE

- Bleeding from one or both nostrils.

Treatment

- Sit patient upright, then blow both nostrils hard to evacuate the clot. Pinch and hold the nose at the nostril crease. Hold constant pressure for fifteen minutes. If unable to control bleeding, consider packing the nose with gauze (soak gauze in regular (non-herbal) tea to assist with constriction of the blood vessels).
- If mild nose bleed that stops on its own, consider applying antibiotic ointment inside nostril to lubricate; otherwise dry skin may be irritated and at risk for rebleeding.

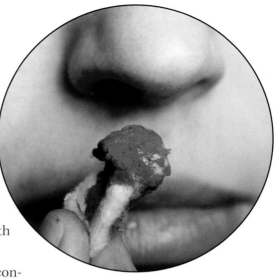

If unable to stop a nose bleed, one option is to pack the nostril with gauze.

SYMPTOMS: THROAT

- Pain to throat, hoarse voice, swollen neck lymph nodes.

Treatment

- Take Motrin, gargle with warm water or salt water.

⚠ **Red Flags:** Pain when opening the mouth, pain to the floor of the mouth or front of the neck, persistent high fevers.

🚁 **Evacuate:**

- Persistent eye pain, purulent discharge, severe redness to both eyes, or any changes in visual acuity to one or both eyes.
- Eye redness/foreign body sensation in a contact lens wearer (which may signify a dangerous infection).
- Impaled object in the eye. Patient will have eyes patched and be unable to see or ambulate. Will need to bring EMS to the patient.
- Persistent nosebleed or nosebleed that requires packing.
- Throat pain with difficulty swallowing, severe pain making it difficult to swallow liquids or food, or a muffled voice.

14

FEMALE GENITAL PROBLEMS

If a woman has a genital problem in the wilderness, diagnosis and treatment is often based solely on a patient's history. It is of primary importance to determine if any female with lower abdominal pain and/or vaginal bleeding is pregnant, as this will necessitate an emergent evacuation to ensure the symptoms are not due to an ectopic pregnancy (an embryo that develops outside the uterus) which is a medical emergency. Severe pelvic pain may be due to twisted ovaries that impinge on the blood supply (torsion), a surgical emergency. Excessive or irregular bleeding may be due to changes in exercise and exertion, and after a negative pregnancy test to ensure no ectopic pregnancy, menstrual flow is best contained with a tampon (if the patient is experienced and comfortable with this technique). Vaginal discharge or itching may be due to humidity and changes in the vaginal flora rather than an infection, and as gynecologic evaluation is unfeasible, any copious discharge or severe pain should be evaluated by definitive medical care.

SYMPTOMS: VAGINAL BLEEDING
- Vaginal bleeding, painful menstrual cramps, bilateral or middle lower abdominal pain, pain two weeks after last menstrual period.

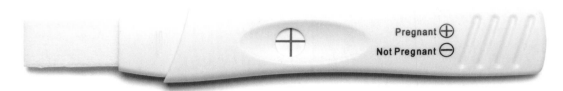

When vaginal bleeding occurs, it is important to determine if the patient is pregnant. This will help determine if evacuation is necessary.

Treatment

- Pregnancy test.
- Motrin or Tylenol (as directed by instruction label) for pain.
- Hot water bottle to abdomen.

SYMPTOMS: URINARY PROBLEMS

- Burning on urination, increased frequency of urination, blood in urine.

⚠ **Red Flags:** Pain and tenderness to flank area and/or fever.

Treatment

- Aggressive hydration.

SYMPTOMS: VAGINAL BURNING, ITCHING, DISCHARGE

Treatment

- Wash vaginal area well, air dry well.
- Consider wearing cotton underwear, especially at night.

SYMPTOMS: PELVIC PAIN

Treatment

- Treat with Motrin every six to eight hours, per the instruction label.

🚁 **Evacuate:**

- Any pregnant patient with lower abdominal pain.
- Severe unrelenting pelvic pain.

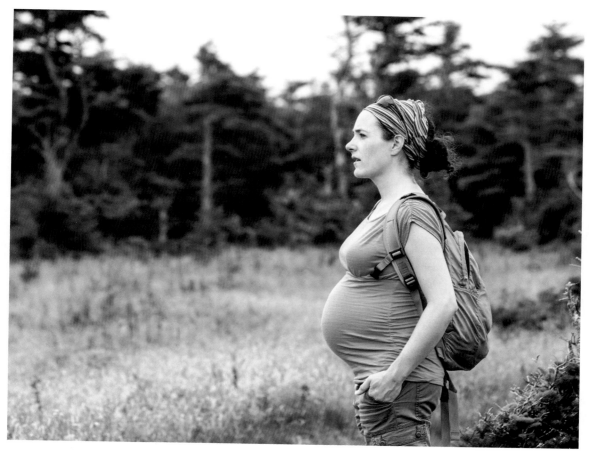

If a pregnant patient has lower abdominal pain or vaginal bleeding, it is best to evacuate.

- Any pregnant patient with vaginal bleeding.
- Symptoms of urinary problems that do not respond to supportive therapy and/or persistent fever, as the patient likely has an infection that will require antibiotics.
- Patient with pain or tenderness to flank area.

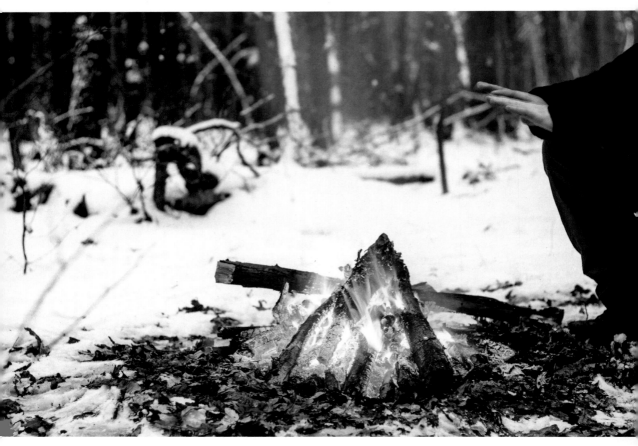

Take steps to keep the extremities warm during freezing weather to avoid frostbite.

15

FROSTBITE

Cold exposure can cause both freezing and non-freezing injuries, depending on the depth of the skin layers involved. Frostnip is ice crystal formation on the superficial layers of skin, not actual skin freezing, and it leads to numb, pale or white soft skin which can be easily treated in the field. Frostbite is the actual freezing of cells that can lead to permanent tissue injury and debilitating outcomes and amputation. Extremities such as ear lobes, nose, fingers, and toes are most prone to cold injury. Factors contributing to cold injury include: hypothermia, prior frostbite, dehydration, constricting clothing/boots, wind, severity of cold environment, and concurrent alcohol or tobacco use (by adults). Cold and wet environments, cold and windy conditions, and extremely low temperatures cause the highest risks for frostbite. Care should be taken to ensure risk awareness in cold weather travelers and that numb extremities are rapidly and repeatedly evaluated for cold injury.

Frostbite typically presents with numbness due to freezing of the nerves along with the other tissue, and the skin's change to a white, waxy appearance, which may become firm or hard depending on the depth of the tissue involved. Rapid rewarming is the mainstay of therapy to decrease tissue loss, unless there is risk of refreezing, as refreezing of the thawed frostbite will cause the injured cells to be further injured, decrease the viability of affected tissue, and worsen outcomes. It is better to hike out on frostbitten toes then to thaw them in the field, and then risk refreezing the injury.

If the decision is made to rewarm frostbite in the field, protect and treat generalized cold injury (*see* **Hypothermia** section), remove constrictive clothing or jewelry, and prepare for a painful situation as the skin is thawed and sensation returns. The injured areas once rewarmed may remain numb, and should be protected against further injury with soft and fluffy bandages if available. Increased pain and bloody blisters or dark dusky skin often occur six or more hours after the initial injury, and reevaluation of the initial frostbite injury may reveal progression and severity of disease.

Frostbite severity is often staged similar to thermal burns and has been also "graded" on appearance of the frostbite lesion post-thawing, however the extent of tissue damage is usually not apparent for several days. As such, one should be conservative in estimating the seriousness of the frostbite injury and assume the worst rather than risk eventual amputation due to initial underestimation.

Grade I: Superficial/partial thickness with resolved lesion or clear blisters, tissue loss is minimal or none, and amputation is rare.

Grade II: Lesions to the distal tips of the fingers or toes.

Grade III: Lesions to fingers or toes up to the knuckle.

Grade IV: Lesions to the mid-foot or hand.

SYMPTOMS

- Pale, white, waxy, hard skin; numbness (may feel like a "chunk of wood").
- Blanching of extremities (pinking of nail bed after pressure takes three seconds or more).
- Blisters (clear).
- Mottled, dusky, "bluish" skin.
- After re-warming, skin is swollen, red, painful.
- May develop clear blisters
- May develop blood-filled blisters (represents a deep tissue injury).

⚠ **Red Flags:** Dusky mottled skin, blood-filled blisters.

Treatment

- Primary treatment is the rapid rewarming of frozen extremity *only* if there is no risk of refreezing.
- Thaw with non-scalding water (104°F–106°F). Water should be hot-tub temperature.
- Keep affected extremity submerged for twenty to thirty minutes, or until skin becomes soft and returns to normal color (likely need to reheat water).
- Motrin (as directed by instruction label) for pain.
- Dress with clean gauze between fingers or toes and around extremity.

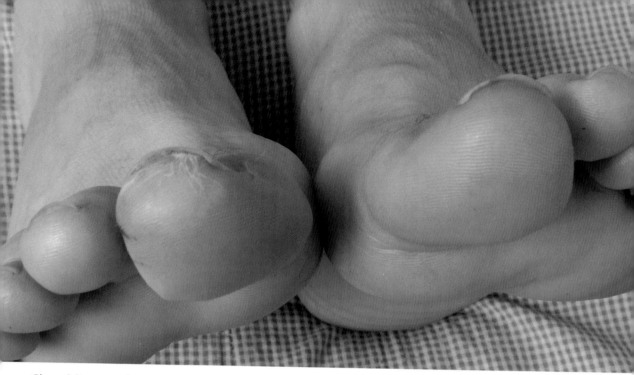

Clear blisters after rewarming are a sign of mild frostbite (Grade I).

- Do not rewarm with radiant heat (fire).
- Do not massage or rub with snow.
- Blisters: drain clear blisters if fluctuant and at risk for spontaneous rupture (*see* **Blisters**). Do not drain blood-filled blisters.

Evacuate:

- Any patient with suspected Grade II to Grade IV frostbite.
- Any patient with blood-filled blisters.
- Any patient with dusky, blotchy skin.
- Any patient unable to use the injured extremity due to either pain or immobility.
- When you are unable to protect area from further cold or refreezing.
- Any patient whose pain cannot be managed in the field.
- When there are any signs of infection to affected area.

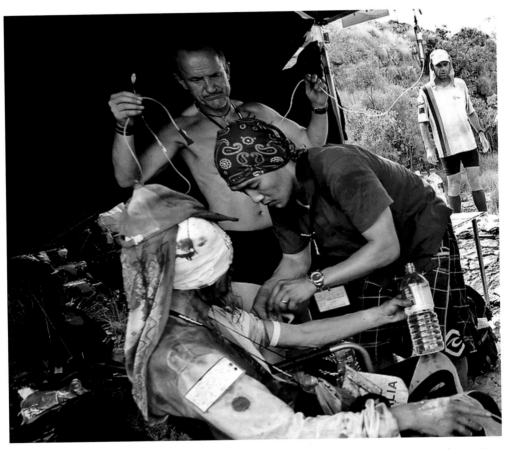

It's important to be vigilant with head injuries, especially during the first twenty-four hours.

16

HEAD INJURY

Anyone who has suffered an injury to the head is potentially at risk for progressive bleeding and swelling in or around the brain. Despite evidence of trauma with scalp bleeding or a large bump or swelling, serious sequalae to most minor head injury is rare. People who have a bleed around their brain deep inside their skull from a head injury may initially appear well and oriented, only to later decompensate with an altered level of responsiveness as the pressure inside the skull increases from the bleeding. The first few hours after a head injury are the most important to observe the patient for worsening symptoms—which may represent a more severe head injury than initially suspected that requires evacuation to medical care and possibly even neurosurgery. Delay in presenting symptoms of a severe head injury are more common in the elderly and children. Be aware of any medications such as anti-platelet drugs or blood thinning drugs (anti-coagulants) that put an individual at higher risk for bleeding and delayed presentations of severe head injury. There is no science that clearly dictates how often someone's neurologic status should be checked to ensure they are not progressing from minor to severe head injury, and if the victim falls asleep, how often they should be woken up to check their status. Immediately following a head injury, someone should not go to sleep as lethargy or somnolence is a concerning sign. But once asleep, it is reasonable to wake them every two to four hours to ensure responsiveness.

Symptoms of a concussion may be present with or without initial loss of consciousness. Always consider the mechanism of injury (MOI) for possible concurrent spinal injury and necessary spinal immobilization precautions. Scalp lacerations tend to bleed, a lot. Apply a wound dressing of gauze folded into a small square over the site of bleeding, as the smaller the surface area of bandage the greater the amount of exerted pressure. Apply compression with a circumferential bandage or compression wrap (*see the* **Wound Care** section for closure of scalp lacerations). Prevention of head injuries should focus on wearing a helmet in high risk situations, like biking, rock climbing, white water sports, or areas with potential for rockfall.

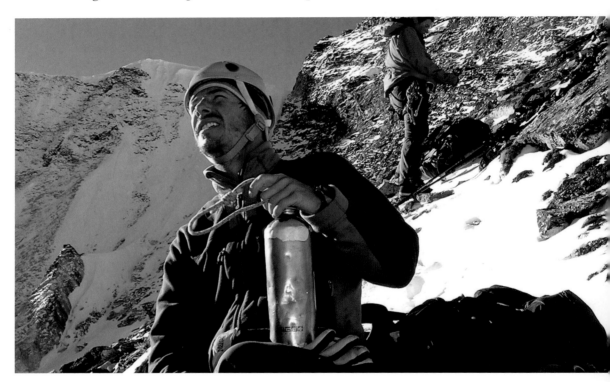

To prevent head injuries, wear helmets during high risk activities. *Credit: Grant Lipman*

SYMPTOMS: MINOR HEAD INJURY

- Headache, transient nausea and/or vomiting, "seeing stars," dizziness, mild decrease in level or responsiveness (LOR), or appears "dazed." These symptoms should resolve quickly.

⚠ **Red Flags:** Loss of consciousness, rapid decompensation after initial injury (patient may appear drunk or have a progressive change in normal behavior).

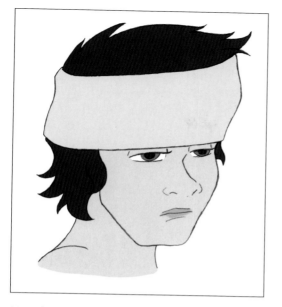

Head injury wrap.

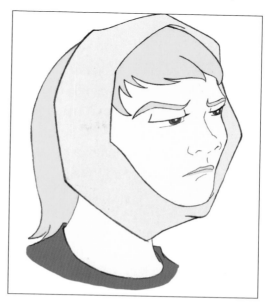

Head injury wrap.

Treatment

- Ensure that symptoms resolve quickly.
- Monitor for twelve hours to ensure no worsening of symptoms.
- Motrin or Tylenol for headache, per the directions on the instruction label.

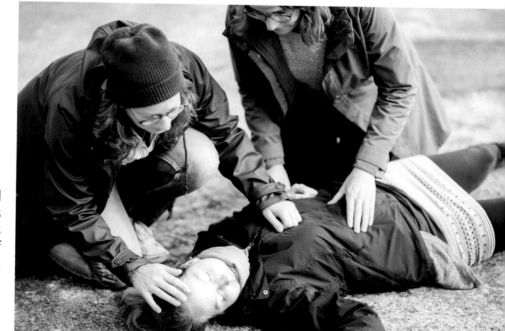

Head injury red flags include loss of consciousness or a lack of responsiveness.

SYMPTOMS: SEVERE HEAD INJURY

- Persistent symptoms of mild head injury that worsen in severity, blurred vision, lethargy, increasing disorientation, irritability, combativeness or otherwise altered level of responsiveness (LOR), persistent sleepiness, lack of coordination, seizures, persistent nausea or vomiting. There may be leaking clear fluid from the nose or ears.

⚠ **Red Flags:** Black eyes or bruising behind ears, worsening symptoms of minor head injury.

🚁 **Evacuate:**

- Any patient with progressive symptoms.
- Any patient with persistent altered LOR after head injury.
- Any patient with symptoms of severe head injury.
- Any patient whose symptoms of minor head injury do not show improvement or persistent or worsening headache after twelve hours.

17
HEAT ILLNESS

Heat illness might be due to passive exposure to high ambient temperatures, overexertion in the heat, under- or over-hydration, or medications that exacerbate the body's response to a hot environment. The hotter the temperature, the more at-risk the patient is to overhydrate, which can be as dangerous (or more so) than dehydration in the heat. Over-hydration with plain water during exertion without eating salty food or consuming electrolytes may lead to a dangerous dilution of the body's salt balance (hyponatremia). Always rehydrate with electrolyte-containing fluids and/or salty foods. Individual risk factors for heat illness include: someone who is not used to hot conditions (unacclimatized), or on certain medications (some cardiac medicines, high blood pressure medicines, anti-anxiety/depressants, over-the-counter cold medicines, alcohol, stimulants). Dehydration will limit the body's ability to respond adequately to heat stress, so always begin exercising in the heat well hydrated.

A person is more susceptible to heat illness in humid conditions, as increased amount of atmospheric water vapor will minimize the vapor pressure gradient between the skin and surrounding air, inhibiting evaporation of sweat and subsequent heat loss. For example, 100°F (37.8°C) in 20 percent humidity will feel like 132°F (55.6°C) in 60 percent humidity. Heat is generated both externally through environmental exposure, and internally through exercise which can increases metabolism by twenty-five times, of which 75 percent to 80 percent is converted to heat. Heat is exchanged through four main mechanisms:

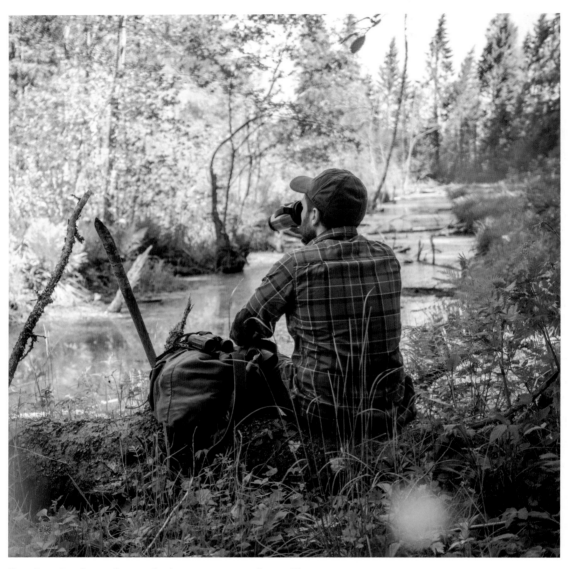

Staying hydrated may help to prevent heat illness.

Convection: Heat transferred through a gas or liquid, like air or water. When the surrounding air is warmer than approximately 91°F (33°C), heat will be gained by the body. Wind chill can cool a body.

Conduction: Heat exchange by two surfaces in direct contact. Immersion in cold water will lose heat; sitting on hot ground (or immersion in hot water) will cause heat to be gained.

Evaporation: As a liquid is phase-changed into a gas, heat is lost. For every 1.7 mL of sweat is evaporated from the skin, 1kCal of heat is lost.

Radiation: Heat transfer through electromagnetic waves. Standing in the sun is a simple example of heat gain through radiation, while the body radiates heat to cool.

Heat illness like swelling to the extremities, muscle cramps ("heat cramps"), or fainting ("heat syncope") are all self-limited. Fainting in the heat is usually due to the heat induced dilation of blood vessels and subsequent pooling of blood in the extremities. The diminished return of oxygenated blood to the brain can cause the dizziness or passing out, which has a spontaneous return to normal level of responsiveness (LOR). Anyone who loses consciousness in the heat has declared themselves poorly acclimatized to the hot conditions, and it is reasonable to observe them for a while, to ensure that they are able to eat, drink, and exert themselves comfortably.

For more severe heat illness, cold water immersion is the fastest and usually only effective way to rapidly cool someone with serious heat illness; immerse up to the level of the armpits and be cautious to keep shoulders and head dry and secure, in case of loss of consciousness. If unable to immerse the patient in a body of water, douse all clothes and head in water to optimize heat transference. Stop the cooling once normal LOR has returned. Be concerned for anyone who is hot with altered consciousness, as this is a heat stroke victim until proven otherwise, which is a life-threatening emergency and they will need to be cooled as rapidly as possible. Altered level of consciousness without elevated body temperature may be hyponatremia, so a careful and accurate patient history of recent fluid consumption and symptoms may be more helpful than a thermometer.

SYMPTOMS: LOW SALT LEVEL (HYPONATREMIA)

- Weakness, nausea, dizziness, headache, fatigue, muscle cramps. May have history of decreased urine output as the body may inappropriately retain water. Symptoms may appear similar to that of heat exhaustion.
- ⚠ Altered LOR (without elevated temperature), seizures, unconsciousness.

Red Flags: Vomiting and unable to tolerate fluids, altered LOR, seizures.

Treatment

- With mild symptoms, stop the patient from further fluid intake and the body will urinate out the excessive fluid balance. Patient should feel better.

- If tolerable, can rehydrate with a concentrated electrolyte solution or salty foods. Can dissolve several bouillon cubes in a cup of water for a highly concentrated salty slurry.
- If any altered LOR or unable to tolerate salty fluids/foods by mouth, evacuate.

SYMPTOMS: HEAT CRAMPS
- Cramps of muscles, which may involve small or large muscle groups.

Treatment
- Stop exertion and rest in shade.
- Gentle stretching and massage to the painful muscles.
- Hydrate with a solution containing electrolytes.

SYMPTOMS: FAINTING
- Dizziness, nausea, loss of consciousness.

⚠ **Red Flags:** Persistent altered level or responsiveness (LOR), inability to eat, drink, or ambulate due to dizziness, concurrent symptoms of chest pain, or shortness of breath.

Treatment
- Stop exertion and rest in shade.
- Rehydrate with electrolyte-containing fluids.
- Evaporative and conductive cooling: wet the victim's clothes/head and make a fan/draft to dissipate heat.

SYMPTOMS: HEAT EXHAUSTION
- Flushed, rapid pulse, sweating, dizzy, nausea, vomiting, muscle cramps, headache, chills, history of decreased fluid intake and/or urine output. May appear with symptoms similar to hyponatremia.
- Crampy abdominal pain.

⚠ **Red Flags:** Dark yellow or bloody urine, decreased urine output, too fatigued to continue, unable to tolerate fluids by mouth.

Treatment
- Stop exertion and rest in shade.
- Aggressively rehydrate with electrolyte-containing fluids.

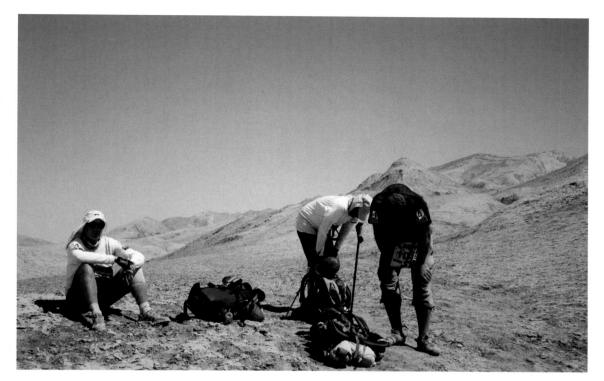

Heat exhaustion can lead to inability to continue exertions and complete immobility.

- Gentle stretching for cramps.
- Evaporative cooling: wet the victim's clothes/head and make a fan/draft to dissipate heat through evaporation.
- Cool with dousing of clothes, head, face, and hands with water.
- If more severe symptoms, can consider immersive cooling.

SYMPTOMS: HEAT STROKE

- Symptoms of heat exhaustion but with altered LOR and elevated temperature.
- Seizure, confusion, unconsciousness.
- Patient may be sweating or have dry skin, may be flushed or pale.

Treatment

- Similar treatment for heat exhaustion, with aggressive cooling: remove constricting and insulative clothing, cold water immersion is first choice (if available), otherwise soak the person all over with available water. Can fan to increase evaporation.

- Cautious hydration of the patient with altered LOR, as they are at risk of seizures and subsequent vomiting and aspiration.
- Cool immediately. Do not delay cooling for evacuating.

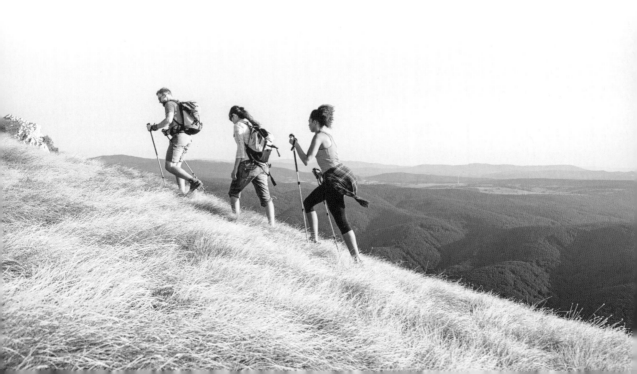

Evacuate:
- Heat stroke (or any altered LOR); these should have EMS brought to them to minimize exertion and further heat generation.
- Persistent symptoms of heat exhaustion that do not improve.
- Red/brown urine.

18
HYPOTHERMIA

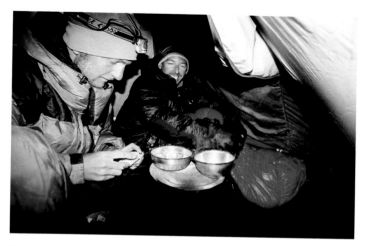

Dress appropriately when out in cold weather to avoid hypothermia and other issues. *Credit: Grant Lipman*

Hypothermia occurs when the body's ability to produce heat through metabolic activity combined with heat retention is overwhelmed by the cold effect. Heat can be lost by the same four mechanisms found in heat illness. Windy and wet conditions lead to more rapid and severe heat loss, with moisture increasing heat loss twenty-four times faster than dry. Hypothermia treatment has three main focuses: (1) to recognize the severity of presenting hypothermia; (2) increase heat production; and (3) minimize further heat loss. Synthetic clothes with multiple layers will be better able to wick sweat and remain warm when wet than organic fibers—hence the saying "cotton kills."

The Swiss have defined the severity of hypothermia (abbreviated HT) based on the presenting signs and symptoms as HT I (mild, clear consciousness with shivering); HT II (moderate, impaired consciousness that may progress to loss of shivering); HT III (severe, unconscious);

HT IV (profound, apparent death); and HT V (death). Cold slows down the body's metabolic processes, with a decrease in brain metabolic rate of 6 percent to 7 percent per 2°F. So someone who is cold with normal mental function may not be hypothermic. Shivering and confusion can further be differentiated from confusion and a lack of shivering in severity of hypothermia. Awareness and recognition of these clinical stages is more important than the patient's temperature, as it may be difficult to obtain an accurate temperature measurement in the wilderness. **HT I:** Mild hypothermia can effectively be managed in the field, but any symptoms of **HT II** or worse (cold and impaired level of responsiveness) must be recognized early, as the wilderness setting offers limited interventions other than providing shelter from the wind and cold, removing wet clothing, and increasing metabolic heat production through exercise and "stoking the fire" through ingesting calories. Recognize that HT II and worse will likely require evacuation and rewarming via hospital care.

Avoid small heat packs for rewarming or body to body contact for hypothermic victims (although useful to warm cold fingers and toes). The localized heating may reduce shivering which will minimize internal heat generation, but they do not appreciably increase the rewarming rate over shivering alone. Calories are more important than a heated drink, as the heat generated from ingested calories will stoke the metabolic furnace and will be more advantageous than a warmed liquid. Consider not walking or exercising the victim for thirty minutes after starting the rewarming process, as this will avoid recirculating the cold blood to the body's core and preventing a precipitous drop in temperature. Be careful and handle HTIII/IV patients gently, as the cold heart is irritable and prone to fatal heart rhythms. Very cold people (especially after cold water drowning) have survived after prolonged arrest, so hypothermia is an exception to the regular instructed time limitations of wilderness CPR. There is a saying, "You are not dead until you are warm and dead," so CPR should be attempted on hypothermic dead-appearing patients, except in situations where there is a non-compressible frozen chest, obvious signs of death (i.e., decapitation) or an avalanche burial longer than thirty-five minutes and airway obstructed with snow.

SYMPTOMS: HT I – MILD HYPOTHERMIA, 95°F–90°F (35°C–32°C)

- Shivering (persistent).
- Loss of fine motor coordination (stumbling).
- Withdrawn, irritability, and poor judgment (mumbling).

Treatment

- Change the environment and find shelter.

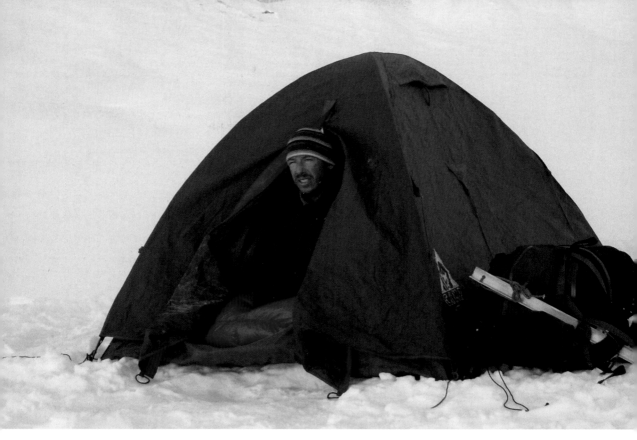

When experiencing mild hypothermia, change your environment or find shelter to escape the cold winds. *Credit: Grant Lipman*

- Replace wet clothing with dry clothing, add wind-resistant and waterproof layers.
- Add insulation under and around the patient.
- Cover head and neck.
- Sweet liquids and food (calories).
- Consider exercise (i.e., calisthenics) to warm up.

SYMPTOMS: HT II – MODERATE HYPOTHERMIA, 90°F–82°F (32°C–28°C)

- Cessation of shivering at approximately 86°F (30°C).
- Altered level of responsiveness (LOR), lethargic, may appear drunk.
- Combative or irrational.
- Slowed heart and respiratory rates.
- Cannot adequately care for themselves.

Treatment

- Evacuate, as unlikely able to increase core temperature.
- Minimize heat loss and cold exposure with maximum insulation and warm hat.
- Be cautious giving fluids or food because of the risk of vomiting and aspiration.
- If in a coma, handle patient gently as heart is prone to fatal heart rhythms.
- Hypothermia wrap if victim is unable to ambulate.

SYMPTOMS: HT III – SEVERE HYPOTHERMIA, 82°F–75°F (28°C–24°C)

- Comatose with fixed and dilated pupils.
- May have rigid muscles.
- Very slow or absent heart rate.

Treatment

- Handle gently.
- Minimize heat loss and cold exposure with hypothermia wrap.
- Evacuate to a hospital with Intensive Care Unit capabilities.

SYMPTOMS: HT IV – PROFOUND HYPOTHERMIA, <75°F (<24°C)

- Likely will appear dead, with very faint or absent vital signs.

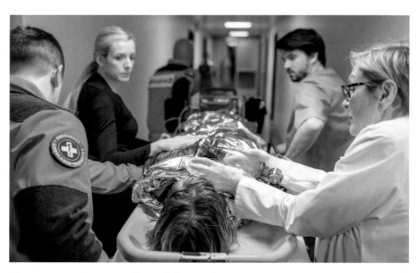

If a patient has profound hypothermia, then it is important to evacuate to a hospital that can adequately treat them.

Treatment

- Handle gently.
- Minimize heat loss and cold exposure with hypothermia wrap.
- Evacuate to a hospital with Intensive Care Unit capabilities.

🚁 **Evacuate:**

- Mild hypothermia (HT I) that is not able to rewarm.
- Moderate and more severe hypothermia (HT II–IV).

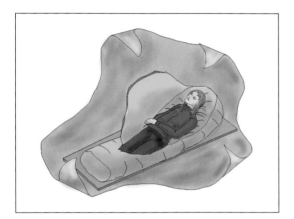 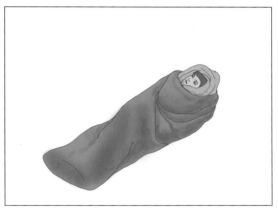

Hypothermia wrap.

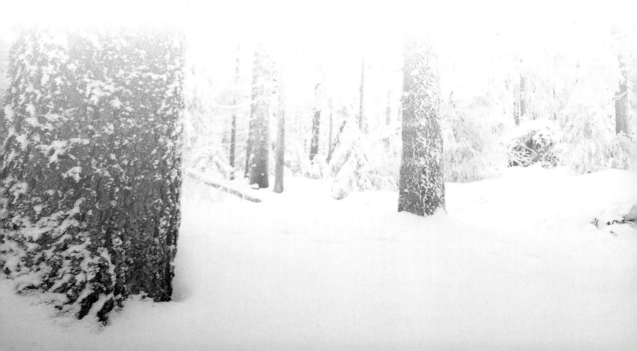

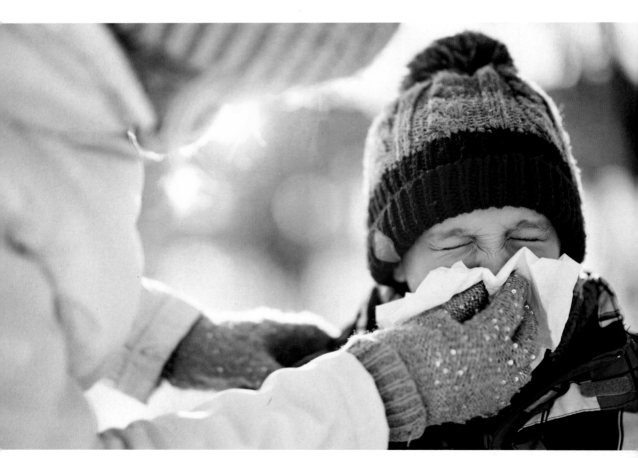

A variety of viral illnesses are common in the wilderness.

19

INFECTIOUS DISEASE

Travel in wilderness areas around the world will expose travelers to diseases unique to that area. Prior to travel, one should check the Centers for Disease Control and Prevention website (www.cdc.gov) for up-to-date emerging infectious diseases and high risk areas around the world. Being outdoors puts one at risk of exposure to mosquito or tick transmitted diseases such as Lyme disease, Rocky Mountain Spotted Fever, Malaria, and Dengue fever, among others. One should be aware of presenting symptoms and signs of indigenous diseases prior to potential exposure.

Viral "flu-like" illnesses are common in the backcountry and may be responsible for a spectrum of symptoms. While most of these symptoms resolve with time (a few days) and symptomatic care, the course of illness may be prolonged and require rest and an evacuation for complete recuperation. Oftentimes, diseases have a delayed presentation due to an incubation period, and diagnostic workup occurs after a wilderness trip has ended. Ticks that have been attached for less than forty-eight hours have very low rates of Lyme disease transmission.

Ensure good hand hygiene before eating and after using the toilet (to minimize the viral spread and/or self-infecting). Do not ingest untreated water. Do not rinse fruit/vegetables in untreated water. Boil water before drinking.

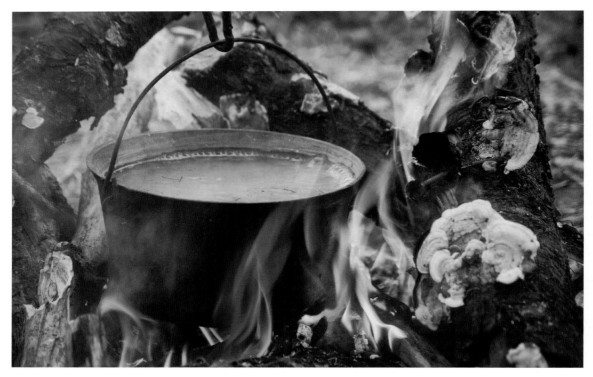

Don't drink untreated water; instead, boil water before use.

SYMPTOMS

- Nausea, vomiting, diarrhea, cough (productive or nonproductive of sputum/mucus), fever, nasal congestion, sore throat, muscle aches, fatigue, headaches.

Treatment

- General management for flu-like illness is treating the symptoms.
- Rest and rehydrate with electrolyte-containing solution. Start slowly (sips every five minutes); then, when the patient is tolerating liquids, aggressively rehydrate with electrolyte-containing fluids.
- Control the nausea with sips of herbal tea, Pepcid and/or Pepto-Bismol as needed (as directed by the instruction label).
- Ibuprofen and acetaminophen for headache, sore throat, muscle aches, per the instructions on the label.

- If frequent diarrhea, Imodium (follow the instructions on the label). Maximum dose is 16mg (eight pills) per day.
- Remove any imbedded ticks with a pair of tweezers, grasping the tick as close to the skin surface as possible. Pull upward gently and with even pressure. Avoid twisting or jerking movements, which can separate tick body or mouth parts which will remain in the skin. Remove any remaining parts, if possible, with tweezers.

Evacuate:
- Fever with headache, stiff neck, and sensitivity to light.
- Flu-like illness with persistent fever and/or difficulty breathing.
- Nausea/vomiting/diarrhea with inability to tolerate fluids for more than twelve hours despite medications.
- A sore throat with inability to swallow water and maintain adequate hydration (feels dizzy on standing and decreased urine output).
- Pale skin, jaundice (yellowed skin), or dark smoky urine.
- High spiking fevers and a non-blanching rash (the rash does not disappear when you press it).

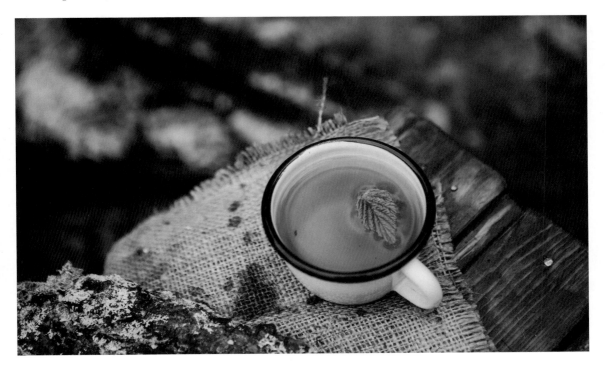

Herbal tea can help manage nausea.

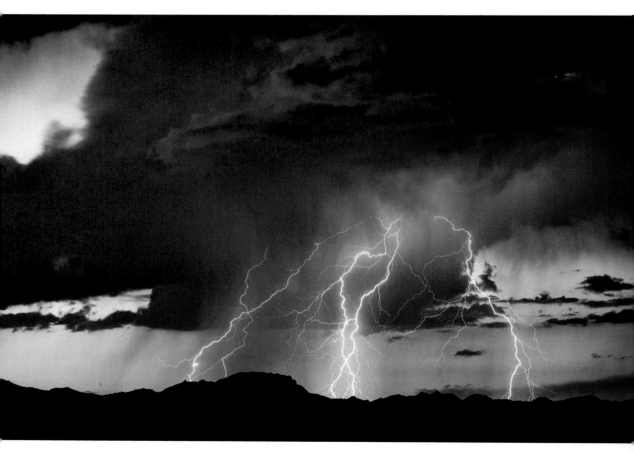

Lightning can be extremely dangerous, so be sure to seek cover.

20
LIGHTNING

Lightning strikes can affect many organ systems in the body including the heart (fatal rhythm), nervous system (bleeding in the brain, seizures, confusion, amnesia, temporary paralysis), the lungs (respiratory arrest), skin (burns), musculoskeletal system (dislocation or fractures, cold and pulseless extremity from blood vessel spasm), and ears and eyes (deafness or blindness).

The victim of a lightning strike may have fixed and dilated pupils, no breathing, no pulse, and may appear dead. However, the rescuer should immediately perform CPR (*see* **CPR**). While CPR in the wilderness usually has a dismal outcome, the massive amount of energy contained in a lightning strike may short circuit the breathing center of the brain and the normal beating rhythm of the heart. While the heart has inherent automaticity and will usually restart spontaneously, the lungs do not have this same ability. Unfortunately the lack of oxygen in this situation will eventually cause the heart to stop beating and the victim will die. So frequent pulse checks during CPR may reveal a heartbeat that has regained a healthy rhythm, but they may need continued assistance with rescue breaths for five or ten minutes until the stunned respiratory center of the brain gets back on-line.

Lightning can strike an individual directly, harm through a concussive blast (from exploding air), or cause injury through side splash (where the lightning jumps from its target to the victim) or through ground current (radiation of the electrical charge through the ground) and conduction. The best treatment is prevention, and awareness of high risk topography, situations, and safest locations can minimize risk.

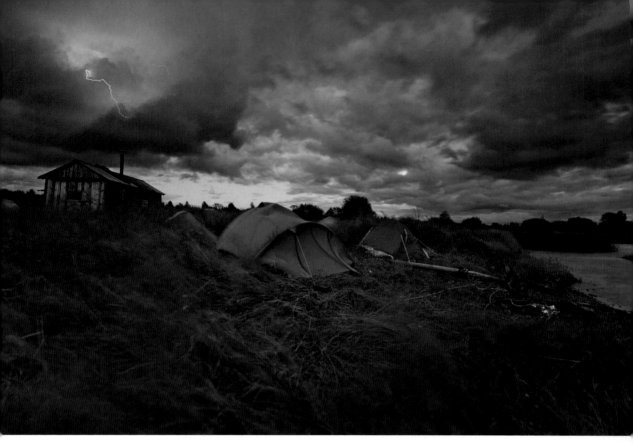

Small shelters like tents are an inadequate shelter during lightning storms.

LIGHTNING PREVENTION

- If time between lightning and thunder is thirty seconds or less, people are in danger of a strike and should seek appropriate cover.
- Wait at least thirty minutes after lightning/thunder before resuming outdoor activity.
- Seek shelter: big buildings, deep caves (three times deeper than wide), metal vehicles.
- Avoid small shelters (e.g., tents), peaks, overhangs, and gullies that may increase risk of ground current injury.
- Avoid contact with metal objects and objects taller than you.
- Do not stand near isolated tall trees (which can injure through side splash).
- Seek a low area near groups of small trees—*not* a clearing where a person may be the tallest object.
- If you are in the open, sit down in a lightning crouch with the legs together to theoretically minimize the voltage difference.

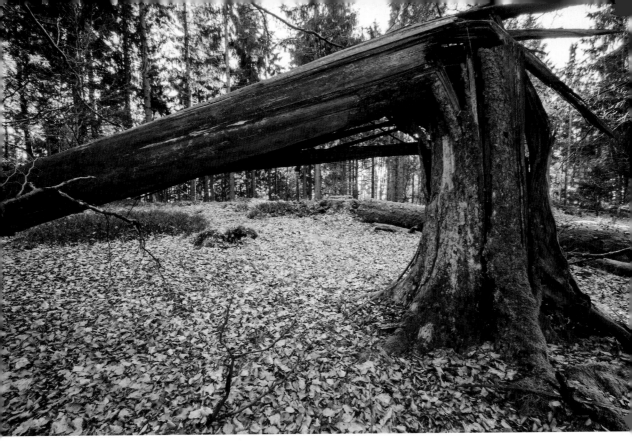

Avoid tall, isolated trees that could fall and injure you during a storm.

- Sit on nonconductive padding (pack, pad, rope, lifejacket).
- If in a group, spread out more than one hundred feet between individuals if possible, while maintaining visual contact (making sure that trip leaders are spread out as well).
- Get out of the water.
- Keep in mind that lightning can strike the same spot twice.
- Lightning in the mountains is more likely in the afternoons.

During lightning storms, avoid being in a clearing or an area where you could be the tallest object.

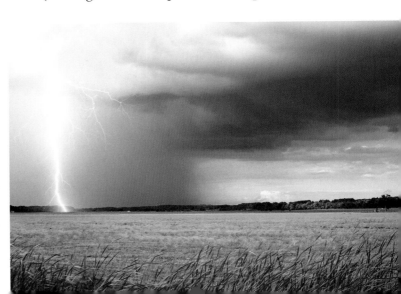

Treatment

- Perform CPR if no pulse. Continue until spontaneously breathing or the rescuer is exhausted.
- If multiple victims require CPR, those with lightning burns to the head have lower rates of survival due to potential devastating brain bleeds.
- Treat injuries as needed.
- Aggressive hydration.

Evacuate: Any patient struck by lightning, with a lightning burn or injury, or unconscious or change in LOR after nearby lightning.

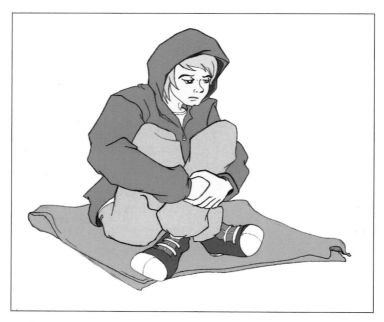

Lightning crouch.

21

LUNG PROBLEMS

There can be many causes for shortness of breath, ranging from minor and non-life threatening issues like anxiety with hyperventilation, to viral infections and inflammatory diseases like bronchitis, to a serious bacterial pneumonia that needs antibiotics, or a medical emergency like a collapsed lung or blood clot. A thorough history will help differentiate the severity of the underlying cause and likely indicate whether an evacuation is necessary.

An infection of the airways or lung tissue is usually from a virus or bacteria. These can both cause high fevers, persistent coughing, phlegm production, and shortness of breath. Treat the fever with Tylenol or Motrin and encourage drinking to combat dehydration. Viral infections often present with associated runny nose, sore throat, muscular aches, and pain. That being said, viruses suppress the immune system, which potentially allows a bacterial infection to worsen. So be suspicious for a secondary infection when someone recovering from a viral syndrome suddenly relapses with a high fever and worsening cough.

A collapsed lung (pneumothorax) can occur from blunt chest trauma or spontaneously in a young healthy person when air escapes from a lung cell, and gets trapped between the chest wall and the lung. The chest pain is sudden, severe, and sharp, and may lead to guarded shallow breaths with shortness of breath. It can be difficult to discern the difference in decreased breath sounds over the area of pain. But if symptoms are worsening or severe, the person should be evacuated. Alternatively, similar symptoms with reproducible tenderness when the chest wall is pushed upon may be a viral infection of the rib lining (costochondritis). This is not associated with shortness of breath, is not serious, and can be treated with Motrin as directed by the instruction label (every six to eight hours as needed).

Similar symptoms as a pneumothorax but more insidious is a blood clot in the lungs (pulmonary embolus). The pain may be dull or sharp, often worse on inspiration, can be increased when lying flat, and associated with shortness of breath, rapid heart rate at rest, and sometimes fever. Pulmonary embolisms are a great mimic for almost any other disease process in the lungs, and risk factors include: birth control, recent prolonged immobility, cancer, and pregnancy, Diagnosis and treatment are only available in a hospital.

SYMPTOMS
- Rapid breathing rate.
- History of asthma or chronic lung disease.
- Audible wheezes.
- Numbness/tingling in the hands and feet.
- Worsening shortness of breath with exertion.
- Chest pain associated with shortness of breath.
- Anxiety.
- Fever and cough with sputum.

⚠ **Red Flags:** Shortness of breath on exertion, or with chest pain. Cough with shortness of breath and/or fever.

Treatment: Anxiety
- If the patient appears anxious with rapid rate of breathing, tingling in hands/feet (suspected anxiety attack), and no history of asthma—calm patient by being direct and reassuring.
- Give sack to breathe into.

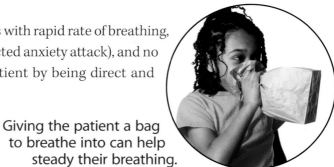

Giving the patient a bag to breathe into can help steady their breathing.

Treatment: Wheeze
- If there is a history of asthma, assist patient with their own medicines (inhaler).
- **Severe:** Gasping with three- to five-word sentences, sweating, may appear fatigued or sleepy. Above medicines and EpiPen to outside of upper thigh. May repeat in five to twenty minutes if initial dose is ineffective or there is a recurrence of symptoms.

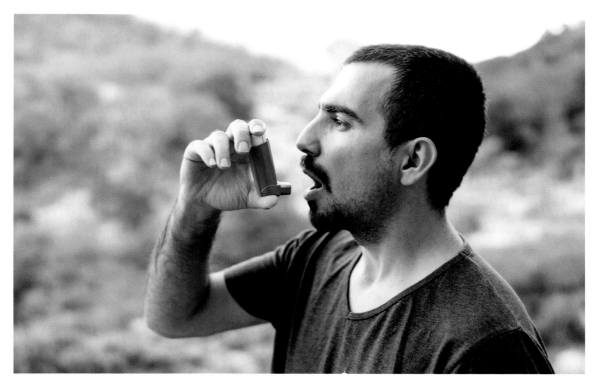

If the patient has an inhaler, using it can help relieve their wheezing.

Treatment: Fever

- Cough with sputum, fever, and worsening shortness of breath, exacerbated by exertion—suspect pneumonia.

Treatment: Chest Pain

- Shortness of breath with chest pain, may be sharp, worse on inhalation, and not reproducible.

Evacuate:

- Asthma attack not responding to the person's inhaler or requiring EpiPen.
- Asthma that does not resolve or worsens despite appropriate medication.
- Cough with fever and worsening shortness of breath.
- Shortness of breath associated with chest pain.
- Shortness of breath that worsens with exertion.

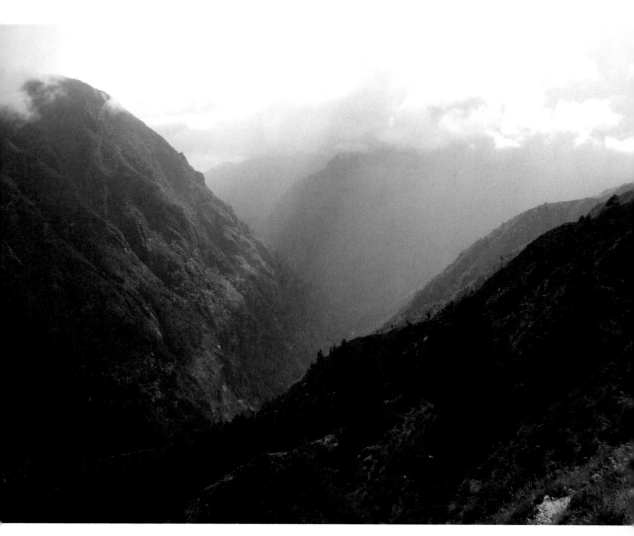

Credit: Grant Lipman

22

MALE GENITAL PROBLEMS

Testicular pain after trauma is the most likely cause of male genital pain in the wilderness—where the severity of pain dictates your ability to manage the situation. If a testicle suddenly becomes painful it may be due to its rotation and twisting on the cord that supplies blood to the scrotum (torsion). This is a surgical emergency and may lead to death of the testicle. If the pain is severe and unrelenting, "detorting" the testicle may resolve the situation while arranging evacuation for definitive care. Some testicular pain can be from an infection. While infectious problems as well as surgical issues will be a challenge to differentiate, delay can result in loss of viability of the testicle so the decision to evacuate for definitive care should err on the conservative side.

SYMPTOMS
- Testicular pain, often one-sided.
- Pain relieved by elevation of the testes
- Hurts to walk or lie flat.

⚠ **Red Flag:** Spontaneous severe testicular pain.

Treatment
- Pain management with Motrin (follow the instructions on the label).
- Cool compress.

- Elevation and support of the testicles.
- Detorting a testes involves grasping it gently and rotating it outwards, like opening a book page. If this worsens the pain, return the teste to its original lie.

Evacuate: Any patient with severe testicular pain.

23

MUSCULOSKELETAL INJURIES

The severity and need for evacuation of a musculoskeletal injury in the wilderness setting will likely be dictated by the ability to use that extremity. For example, a twisted ankle that is too painful to walk on may require a similar treatment of immobilization in the field and subsequent evacuation as a broken ankle. If the injury is a direct blow or fall, always consider a broken bone. If the injury is from a twisting motion, a sprain or strain is most common. A sprain and strain are injuries to the rubber band–like connective tissues (ligaments and tendons) attaching the bones and muscles to each other. Depending on the severity of the tear to these tissues, there may be bruising, swelling, or joint instability. Look at the uninjured extremity to compare deformity, angulation, and overall appearance. Immobilization of the injured area will decrease pain by limiting movement.

Sometimes overuse of an extremity can lead to inflammation, swelling, and pain without an acute injury. The pain and swelling from an overuse injury can be severe, and while usually not serious can potentially be debilitating. For example, a snow shoeing trip with severe Achilles tendinitis would be miserable. Likewise, forearm tendonitis or shoulder or elbow bursitis while canoeing could end the activity. An anti-inflammatory like Motrin and rest can improve the pain.

Dislocations result in an oddly shaped joint that cannot be normally ranged. The most common dislocations are the shoulder, finger, ankle, and patella (knee cap). Any dislocations may be associated with a broken bone. Consider reducing a dislocation in the field if you have specific training in the technique and if the patient is amenable to an attempt. In general, both the difficulty of reduction and the amount of long-term complications increase

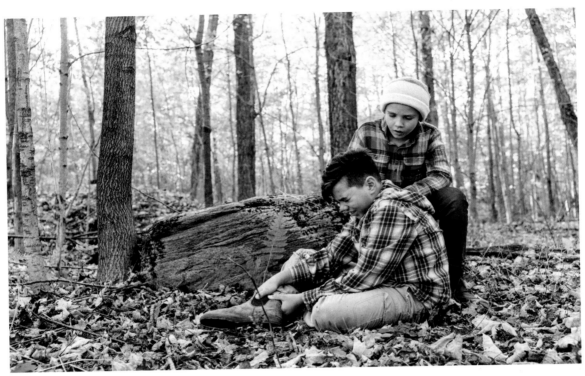

A twisted ankle can be severe enough to limit mobility.

with delay in reduction attempts. Always check CSM—**circulation** (healthy pinking of the nail bed after pressure should take less than three seconds), **sensation** (dull versus sharp differentiation), and **movement** of the joint—and note the status and any change after the reduction attempt. All dislocation/reduction attempts should be performed with a calm and reassuring voice, applying slow, gentle, and constant effort. Avoid sudden jerky movements which can increase the individual's pain, and decrease both the ability to overcome resistant muscle spasm as well as the victim's willingness to allow a second attempt if initially unsuccessful. If pain or resistance, go slower (think of the reduction movement like a minute hand on a clock, rather than the second hand), while maintaining constant force and calming voice.

SYMPTOMS: BROKEN BONE
- Angulation or movement where no joint exists ("a false joint").
- Point tenderness on the bone.
- Inability to bear weight.

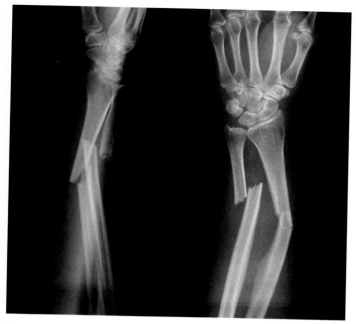

X-ray of a broken arm.

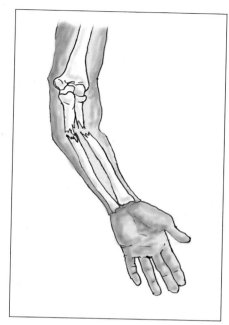

Angulation.

- Hear or feel the grinding of bones together.
- Swelling or discoloration at the point of pain.

⚠ **Red Flags:** Loss of CSM, angulation, or severe tenderness to a bony point.

Treatment

- Remove jewelry.
- Pad bony points with soft material.
- If weight bearing/usable, suspect a sprain/strain and apply compressive bandage wrap.
- If not weight bearing or patient is unable to use extremity, suspect broken bone and apply sling or rigid splint (SAM splint).
- Sling/Splint: Immobilize joint above and below injured site in natural position.
  - ➤ **Wrist:** Splint in position like holding a beverage can (SAM splint).
  - ➤ **Ankle/Elbow:** Splint in 90-degree flexion (SAM splint/sling/sleeping pad). Secure firmly but not tightly.
  - ➤ **Collarbone:** Immobilize the affected extremity with a sling, and may further minimize movement and pain with a swathe (a circumferential bandage around both the upper arm and the trunk).

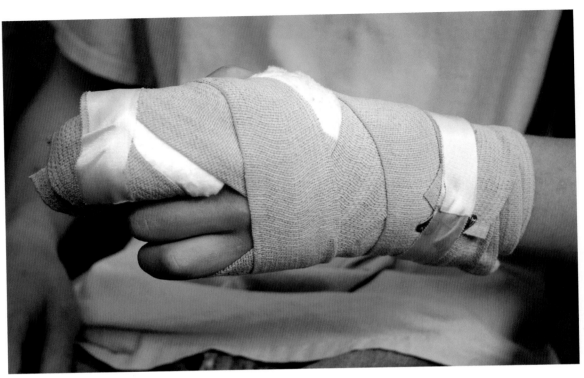

Broken fingers can be taped together.

> **Fingers:** Broken fingers can be buddy taped together.
> **Rib fractures:** Wrap a compression wrap or similar wide bandage circumferential-ly around the fractured ribs to effectively buddy tape them to the uninjured neigh-boring ribs. Encourage the person to take deep breaths to minimize collapse of compressed lung tissue and subsequent infection.
> **Lower leg:** Rigid splint on either side, or behind the injured area. A sleeping bag can be wrapped around the injured part like a burrito and secured with tape. Make sure to put padding in the fossa behind the knee.

- Motrin or Tylenol as needed, and per the instruction labels.
- Check CSM before and after splint application.
- If open bone, irrigate copiously with drinkable water, then cover with antibiotic ointment and sterile/clean gauze.

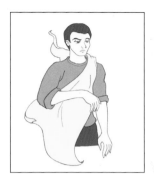 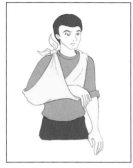 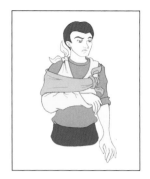 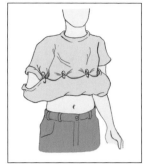

Sling from fabric or triangular gauze.

Improvised sling with safety pins.

SYMPTOMS: SHOULDER DISLOCATION

- Loss of natural curve of shoulder (shoulder appears squared).
- Holding affected arm up and away from body.
- Unable to touch unaffected (opposite) shoulder with the fingers of the injured arm.

Note: Only attempt reductions if trained in the procedure *and* patient is amenable.

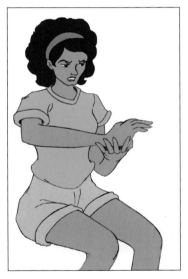 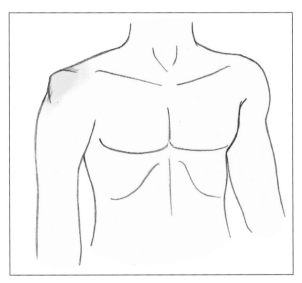

Body position of a dislocated shoulder.

Appearance of dislocated shoulder.

Treatment

- Remove jewelry.

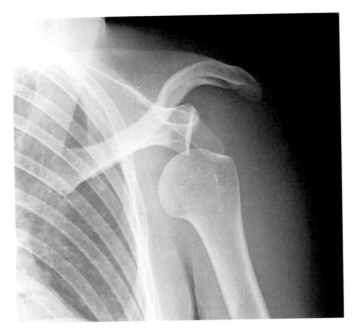

X-ray of a dislocated shoulder.

- Assess CSM.
- Reduce dislocation.
- If successful reduction, you may feel or hear a "thunk" and significant resolution of the individual's pain.
- Recheck CSM and sling arm.

Knee-Wrap Self-Reduction Technique:

- Sit the injured person down with bent knees.
- Clasp both their hands around knees and have them lean back, *slowly* inducing constant traction to overcome the shoulder muscle spasm until the shoulder reduces.

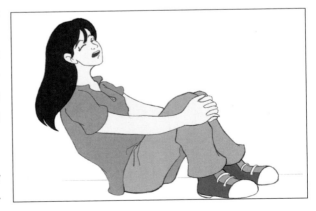

Shoulder reduction by knee-wrap technique.

Tree-Hug Reduction Technique:

- Have the injured person wrap their arms around a slender tree (hugging it).
- Clasp both their hands around trunk and have them lean back, *slowly*, putting all their body weight into it, until the constant traction overcomes the shoulder's muscle spasm and the shoulder reduces.

Spaso Reduction Technique:

- Have the injured person lie on his back, relaxing the shoulder to allow the shoulder blade to rest on the ground, and with calm and gentle voice and movements, grasp the injured arm by the wrist, holding straight up (perpendicular to the body).
- Apply gentle vertical traction for a few minutes while holding the arm straight.
- Keep patient relaxed while doing this, so the shoulder blade stays flat and in contact with the ground.
- Apply gentle external rotation (rotate toward the thumb side of the hand).
- After a few minutes of traction, reduction should occur.

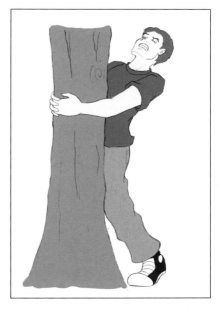

Shoulder reduction by tree-hug technique.

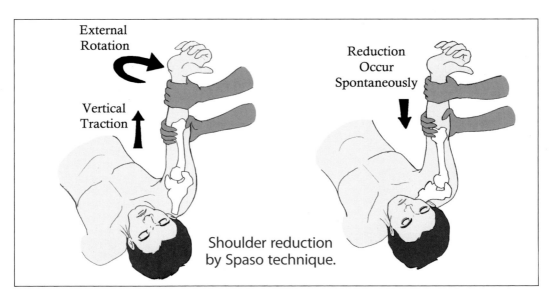

External Rotation

Vertical Traction

Reduction Occur Spontaneously

Shoulder reduction by Spaso technique.

External Rotation Technique*:

- Have injured person lie on his or her back, and with calm and gentle voice and movements, have them bend their affected elbow at 90 degrees.
- Holding affected arm above and at the elbow, bend the shoulder to 90 degrees, which will slowly bring the arm out and away from body.
- Angle the point of the elbow towards the rib cage (which will tilt the arm upwards and outwards).
- Rotate arm outward like opening a book (so back of hand and forearm are facing the ground).
- If necessary, from the open book position, you can bring the arm up (to end up in a position similar to an overhand throw), at which point reduction should occur.
- Be patient, as this process may take five to ten minutes. If resistance is met or pain increases, slow or stop movement, holding position until pain is overcome.

* This technique can be performed with the injured person sitting upright with a straight back, ideally against a vertical support.

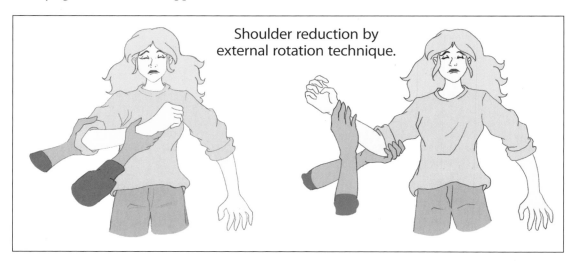

Shoulder reduction by external rotation technique.

SYMPTOMS: KNEECAP DISLOCATION

- Knee feels unstable/leg collapsed.
- Kneecap is repositioned to the outer aspect of the leg.

Treatment

- Sit patient up, flexed at hip, making a 90-degree angle with the leg and torso.
- Straighten leg while pushing kneecap toward the midline (with continuous rapid motion).
- Hyperextend leg (bend the knee opposite of natural joint movement). Knee cap should pop back in.
- Post-reduction patient can weight bear and walk out.
- Immobilize knee with sleeping pad/rigid splint (fashion "suspenders" to keep pad from slipping if needed).

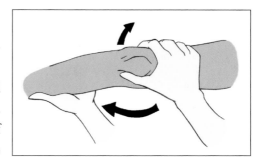

Kneecap reduction.

SYMPTOMS: FINGER OR TOE DISLOCATION

- Fingers angulated at a joint.
- Unable to bend finger joint.

Treatment

- Slow steady movement.
- Do not jerk.
- Holding the injured digit partially flexed, pull on the end towards the angle of the dislocation (pull the direction the finger or toe is pointing in).
- Pull until you hear a "pop" and joint appears to have normal orientation.
- Buddy-tape finger or toe (with adjacent finger or toe).

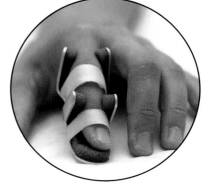

Use a splint to immobilize and splint the finger or toe dislocation.

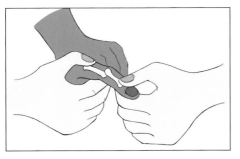

(Left) Finger reduction.

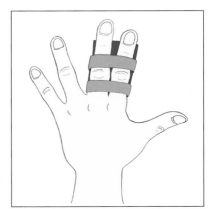

(Right) Finger buddy-taping.

SYMPTOMS: ANKLE DISLOCATION

- Angulation (often pointing outwards from midline).
- Bony protrusion/tenting of skin.
- Pain and inability to weight bear.

Treatment

- Have the injured person lie down with affected leg bent at the knee.
- Have one person hold and stabilize the lower leg at the calf (for counter-traction, providing an anchor).
- Have the second person grasp mid-foot just below the ball of the foot (one hand) and at the heel (second hand).
- Applying constant strong force, pull away from body in direction foot is pointing (traction).
- Once a release of tension is felt, guide foot back to midline.
- Check CSM and splint.

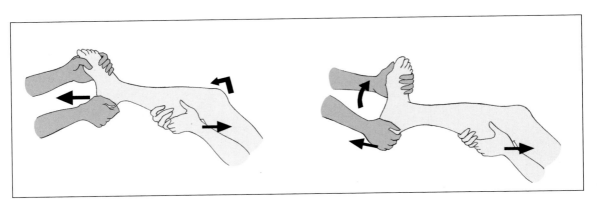

Ankle reduction technique.

Evacuate:

- Any patient with an unreduced dislocation.
- Any patient with altered CSM before or after reduction.
- Any *unusable* musculoskeletal injury, whether a suspected sprain, strain, broken bone, or dislocation. Either due to pain or joint instability.

24
NERVOUS SYSTEM

Injury to the brain from a blood clot or bleeding in a vessel can present as many different symptoms, depending on the area and amount of tissue involved. Strokes can cause symptoms (neurologic deficit) that impair speech, vision, motor function, sensation, balance or coordination, level of consciousness, of even the ability to breathe. Strokes are sudden, with weakness or numbness that typically involve one side of the body, can be either transient or constant, and may be associated with a severe "thunderclap" headache.

Patients with known seizure disorder (epilepsy) are usually on prescription medicine to control their seizures. Ideally, they should have their seizures well controlled by medicine or be seizure free for at least six months, carry their own medicine, and be cleared by their medical doctor before embarking into the wilderness. Seizures can occur as a primary disorder (i.e., epilepsy) or secondary to an environmental injury or other illness (e.g., low blood sugar, low salt level, heat stroke, head trauma, stroke, etc.). If the patient does not have a known diagnosis of epilepsy, look for potentially reversible causes.

SYMPTOMS: NEUROLOGIC DEFICIT
- Decrease in muscle strength or sensation on one side (face, arm, and/or leg).
- Unsteady gait.
- Dizziness.
- One-sided facial droop.

- Severe thunderclap headache.
- Bilateral leg weakness/numbness progressing up the body.

⚠ **Red Flags:** Any neurologic deficit or change in level of responsiveness (LOR).

Treatment
- Place the patient in a position of comfort unless unconscious, then position patient in the recovery position.
- Thorough physical exam to document neurologic deficits and any changes.

SYMPTOMS: SEIZURE
- Patient feels encroaching seizure (aura).
- Blank staring gaze for few seconds.
- Involuntary movement of a localized extremity without loss of consciousness.
- Generalized shaking of entire body with unconsciousness.
- Incontinence of bowel/bladder.
- Altered level of responsiveness (LOR) post-seizure.

⚠ **Red Flags:** Any seizure in a person without known epilepsy (first-time seizure). Multiple seizures or prolonged duration than usual.

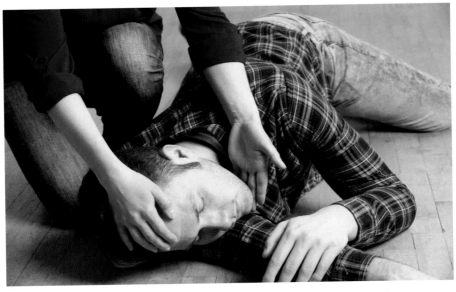

After a patient stops seizing, move them into recovery position.

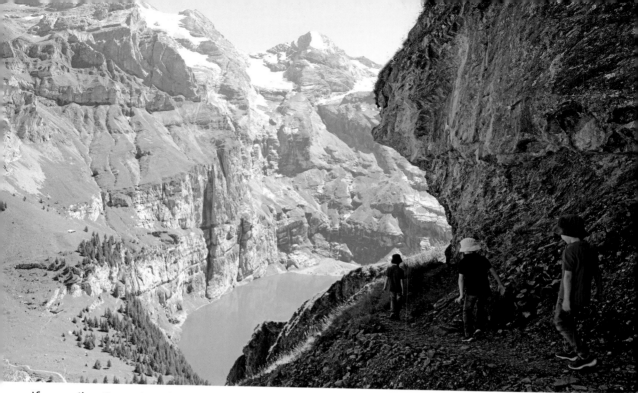

If an epileptic patient just recovered from a seize, do not bring them into hazardous terrain, such as narrow cliffs.

Treatment

- Protect patient (move patient away from environmental hazards).
- Place pad under head if generalized seizure.
- If patient appears to be choking or turns blue, use head tilt/jaw thrust maneuver to open airway. Never put your finger or another object in a seizing person's mouth.
- Once recovered, position patient in recovery position.
- Perform complete physical exam to check for injuries.

Evacuate:

 • Any patient with a focal neurologic deficit.

- Any new seizure.
- Patient with epilepsy, who has multiple seizures without regaining consciousness, or a prolonged seizure over fifteen minutes.
- Any epileptic on trip who has had a simple seizure and is now going into potentially hazardous terrain (e.g., narrow cliff hike, kayaking, etc.).
- Any patient with an altered level of responsiveness (LOR) of unknown origin.

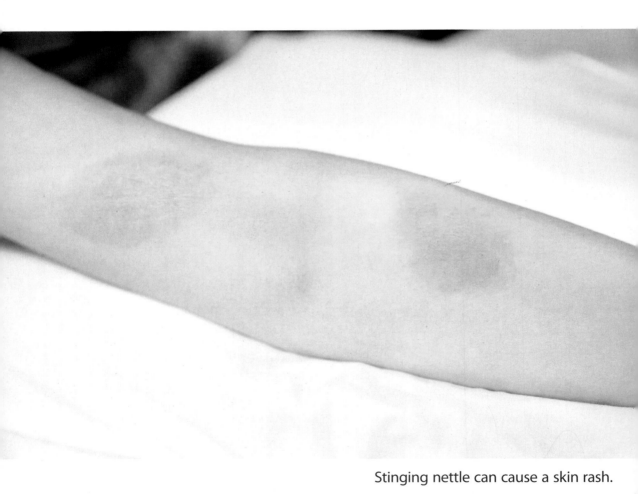

Stinging nettle can cause a skin rash.

25

SKIN IRRITATION

The skin can be irritated from a resin (urushiol) found in the sap of certain plants. The most common toxic plants are poison oak, poison ivy, stinging nettles, and poison sumac that causes a toxic reaction to the skin (contact dermatitis). Poison ivy can appear as a shrub, or grow to a tree size with reddish leaves when young or dark red green leaves when older. Like poison oak, remember, "leaves of three, let it be." Post-exposure, a thorough washing of the exposed skin with soap and water is necessary to remove the resin, as it is irreversibly bound to the skin within thirty to sixty minutes. Individuals have different sensitivities to urushiol, with a reaction that can occur within eight hours to as long as three weeks. The resin can be spread on clothing, camping equipment, or the fur of pets; and last for years if not washed off. Red, swollen, and irritated skin with lines of small blisters are the classic presentation. The blister fluid is not contagious, and the body's immune reaction can cause rash and blisters on parts of the skin that were not exposed. Inhaled smoke from burning plants can also cause a reaction to the nose, mouth, and throat.

A bacterial infection of the skin (cellulitis) presents as spreading redness, warmth, pain, and may have collections of pus (abscess). The redness can be raised, swollen, and confluent, or linear streaks. There may be an associated fever. Any

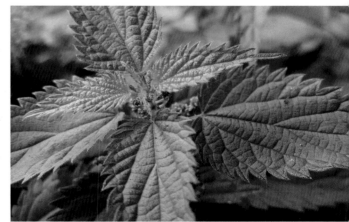

Learn to identify toxic plants such as poison oak.

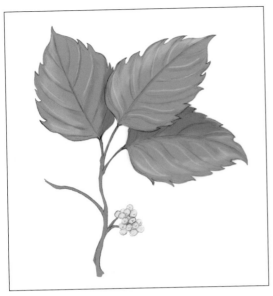

Poison ivy.

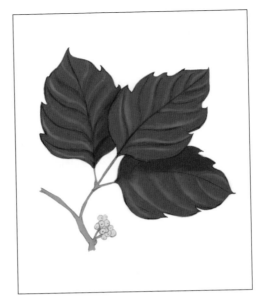

Poison oak.

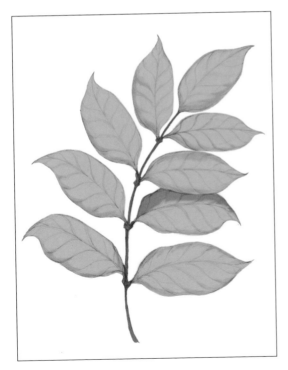

Poison sumac.

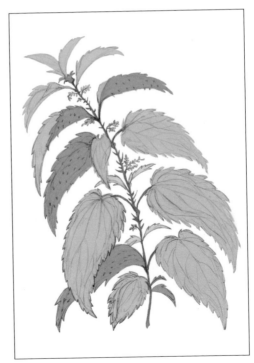

Stinging nettle.

concerning signs of a bacterial infection will require evacuation for medical evaluation and antibiotics.

SYMPTOMS

- Itchy red rash, fluid-filled blisters. Skin irritation may be delayed for up to three weeks.

Treatment

- Wash the affected area (or suspected exposed area) well with soap and water, ideally within thirty minutes of exposure.
- Wash all clothes and equipment that may have been exposed.
- Once the rash appears, itching can be relieved with hydrocortisone cream. More severe itching can be treated with oral Benadryl (follow the instructions on the label).
- Severe blistering may need a two-week prescription steroid (prednisone).

Evacuate:

- Any reaction that involves the eyes, genitals, airway, or breathing.
- Skin irritation that is too uncomfortable to continue trip.
- Any signs of infection to skin (e.g., spreading redness, warmth, and/or pus).

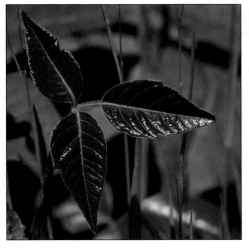

Poison ivy.

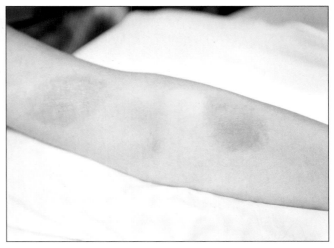

A rash caused by poison ivy or other toxic plants can be relieved with Hydrocortisone cream.

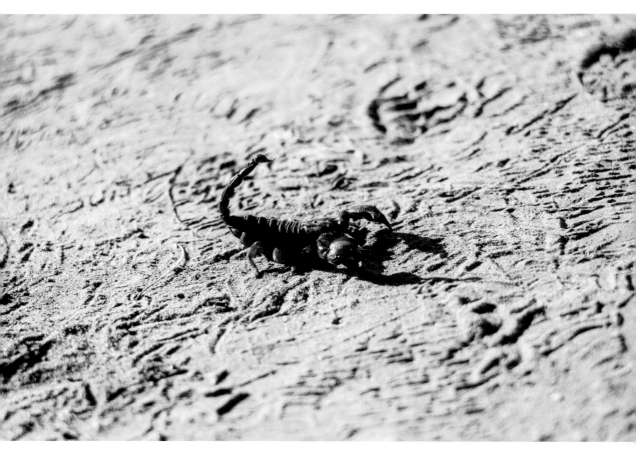

A bark scorpion. All scorpion stings are cause for immediate evacuation.

26

TOXINS, BITES, AND STINGS

The effects of a toxin from a bite or sting from an animal or insect can range from a mild local reaction to a critical life-threatening situation. The most concerning toxin in North America is from a snakebite. There are two types of venomous indigenous snakes, the pit vipers (e.g., rattlesnakes, water moccasins, copperheads) and coral snakes. Most injuries are from pit vipers. Approximately 25 percent of pit viper bites are "dry bites," and do not result in envenomation. However, as symptoms and signs of envenomation may be delayed for up to six to eight hours, and the definitive treatment is antivenin, all snakebites should be evacuated for observation in a hospital setting. If the victim is more than a few hours from a hospital, walking the person out on their own (at the risk of increasing circulation of the toxin) may be more expeditious to decrease the time getting to antivenin, than going for a rescue.

Typical signs of a pit viper envenomation are severe burning pain at the bite site (two puncture wounds), swelling and bruising around the bite area that spreads towards the center of the body, difficulty breathing and rapid heart rate, weakness, and collapse. Fatalities within minutes of a snakebite is very rare, and usually due to anaphylaxis (*see* **Allergic Reaction**). Most coral snakes are found in the Southeast or Southwest United States. These have a neurotoxin, which have a rapid onset and present with numbness, weakness, vomiting, drooling, slurred speech, difficulty breathing, altered level of responsiveness (LOR), and collapse.

IF BITTEN BY A SNAKE:

- Do NOT panic. Calm down the victim, offer reassurance, and plan the evacuation.
- Avoid further injuries. Most snakebites are defensive strikes, so keeping a distance of at least the length of the snake should be safe.
- Attempt to identify the snake with a picture. Do NOT attempt to capture the snake as that may result in an additional victim.
- Do NOT place a tourniquet. This could cause further tissue damage to the underlying skin and muscle already made fragile from the destructive toxins.
- Place a splint to immobilize the extremity if not using that extremity to self-evacuate.
- Do NOT place ice on a wound.
- Do NOT apply a Sawyer extractor pump (they don't help, they just suck).
- If bitten by a coral snake and trained in the application, use the pressure-immobilization technique.

The black widow spider found in North America has a bite that can cause significant injury. The female black widow is a glossy black with a red dot or hourglass shape on its back. Its bite is felt like a pinprick, and severe painful muscle spasms usually begin within the hour and can progress in intensity and include vomiting and difficulty breathing. It may be more severe for a pregnant woman or child. Symptoms are treated with pain medicine and usually resolve within one to two days. There is an anti-venom reserved for severe envenomations.

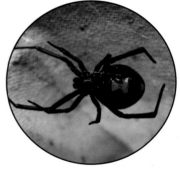

A black widow spider. *Credit: Shenrich91, CC BY-SA 3.0*

In North America, the one scorpion which has a dangerous sting is the bark scorpion (see image on page 272), found in the dry desert habitats of the Southwest. This small yellowish-brown scorpion has a sting that causes immediate burning pain, which is exacerbated by tapping on the site. There is potential for progression of systemic and neurologic symptoms including: sweating, drooling, muscle spasms, seizures, and breathing difficulties and collapse. As symptoms are progressive and may require intensive care unit medical support, all scorpion stings should be evacuated.

Ingested plants and berries found in the wilderness may cause dangerous toxicities. Similar to overdoses of drugs or medicines, the inciting agent may be difficult to identify. Regardless, the goals of treatment are the same: minimize exposure, dilute (if possible), and maximize excretion of the toxin. Give symptomatic support, as specific antidotes are unlikely to be available in a wilderness environment.

SYMPTOMS: SNAKEBITE

- Oozing at site, significant pain from bite, swelling, bruising, discoloration.
- Possible shortness of breath, wheezing.
- Possible numbness to mouth or tongue, muscle weakness, collapse.

⚠ **Red Flags:** Any swelling or skin discoloration, severe persistent pain at bite site, or any neurologic symptoms indicates envenomation.

Treatment

- Remove constricting clothing and jewelry.
- Clean area and dress wound with antibiotic ointment.
- Mark site of initial bruising/swelling by circling with a pen.
- If difficulty breathing/wheeze, treat like anaphylaxis (*see* **Severe** in the **Allergic Reaction** section).
- Evacuate all victims of snakebites.

🚁 **Evacuate:**

- All snakebites, regardless of swelling or bruising, as symptoms may progress over the next six to eight hours.
- Ambulate if able (as minimal time to an emergency room is the most important consideration), otherwise send for assistance.

SYMPTOMS: SPIDER BITE

- Pin prick or painless bite.
- Severe muscle cramps and pain in bitten extremity.
- May involve stomach or chest muscles, vomiting, difficulty breathing, blistering or redness to site.

Treatment

- Clean bite with soap and water.
- Ibuprofen or Tylenol as needed for pain, per the instructions on the labels.
- Apply cold compress to area.

🚁 **Evacuate:**

- Severe pain within sixty minutes of bite.

- Any systemic symptoms.
- Any black widow spider bite.

SYMPTOMS: SCORPION STING

- Painful sting, burning pain to site, numbness to site, positive "tap test," paralysis, muscle spasms, blurred vision, difficulty swallowing, slurred speech. breathing problems.

Treatment

- Apply cool compress to site.
- Ibuprofen or Tylenol as needed for pain, per the instructions on the label.

Evacuate: All scorpion stings. Symptoms may progress over six to eight hours. Evacuate early.

SYMPTOMS: INGESTED TOXIN

- Mild nausea, vomiting, diarrhea, headache, collapse, seizures.

Treatment

- Remove patient from offending toxin (i.e., tent with stove possibly causing carbon monoxide toxicity).
- Treat nausea and vomiting with sips of herbal tea and Pepcid (as directed by instruction label).
- If absorbed toxin, wash off area with soap and water.
- If able, contact the American Association of Poison Control Centers (1-800-222-1222).

Evacuate:
- Inability to tolerate fluids.
- Persistent weakness due to vomiting.
- Collapse.

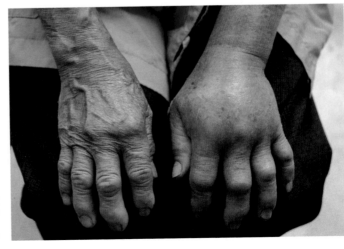

Swelling or bruising at the site of a snakebite is a red flag and cause for evacuation.

SYMPTOMS: STINGS OR BITES (INSECTS, BEES, WASPS, ANTS, TICKS)

- Local pain, swelling, redness, weakness, nausea, vomiting, fever.
- Allergic reaction.

Treatment

- Scrape off stinger.
- If tick is imbedded, grab the head with tweezers as near to the skin as possible, and with constant gentle force, pull up and away.
- Wash area well with soap and water.
- Cold compress to area.
- Benadryl (as directed by the instruction label) for local inflammation/itching (*see* **Allergic Reaction**).
- If wheezing or difficulty breathing, treat for anaphylaxis.

🚁 **Evacuate:** Any sting with associated breathing difficulties or severe allergic reaction/anaphylaxis.

SYMPTOMS: JELLYFISH

- Skin irritation, severe burning, itching, nausea and vomiting, headache, muscle aches, dizziness, numbness, seizure, collapse, altered level of responsiveness (LOR).

Treatment

- Rinse wound with sea water (avoid fresh water).
- Rinse with vinegar (avoid vinegar if suspected Portuguese man-of-war).

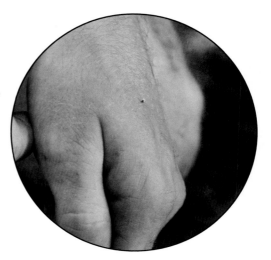

If stung by an insect, begin treatment by removing the stinger.

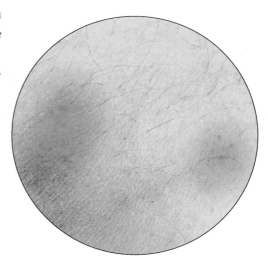

Taking Benadryl can help reduce the inflammation and itching from a bug bite.

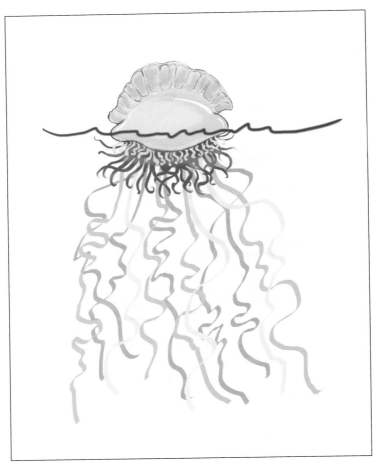

Portuguese man-of-war jellyfish.

- Make a paste of sand and water; scrape off extra stinging cells with edge of card/knife.
- Apply hot water after stinging cells have been scraped off.
- If allergic reaction or anaphylaxis, treat accordingly.

Evacuate: Severe pain, any severe allergic reaction, or any breathing problems or neurologic problems.

27
TRAUMA

The first premise in evaluating any trauma victim is to ensure that the scene is safe for the rescuer; otherwise good intentioned assistance may lead to a second victim. Rock fall, animal attack, thin ice, or a fast river, for example, must all be taken into consideration *prior* to approaching a hurt individual. Always consider the mechanism of injury (MOI) that may have injured the spine, and if concerning, the hurt individual should be kept still with the rescuer's hands while evaluating potential injuries. Damage to the spinal cord can cause permanent paralysis or death. Damage to the bones in the neck (cervical spine) can paralyze the body's ability to breathe. So proper care and management of the suspected spinal injury may prevent an injury to the bones around the spinal cord damaging the underlying nerves.

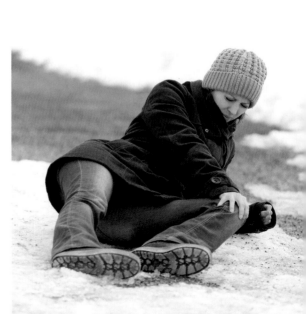

Considering the mechanism of injury—such as slipping on ice—can increase awareness of a potential spinal cord injury and avoid further damage.

TRAUMA BEST PRACTICES

- Take *early* spinal precautions with patients prior to the **Focused Assessment of Cervical Spine (FACS).**
- Always ensure good breathing and a clear airway first.
- If a second rescuer is available, have them hold the cervical spine stable.
- Assume there is a spinal injury if a patient has altered level of responsiveness (LOR) or is unconscious.
- If it's necessary to roll a person (log roll) or move them to a safer environment, the movement should be coordinated by the rescuer at the head, ensuring the rolling/moving is done as a unit with as little angulation or side-to-side movement as possible.
- Ask the victim if there is any spine or back midline pain, weakness, or numbness to hands or feet prior to examination.
- Feel along the entire spine, looking for midline tenderness.
- If the person is conscious and reliable, the utilization of the **FACS** can determine the presence or absence of a bony injury that could cause spinal cord compromise.

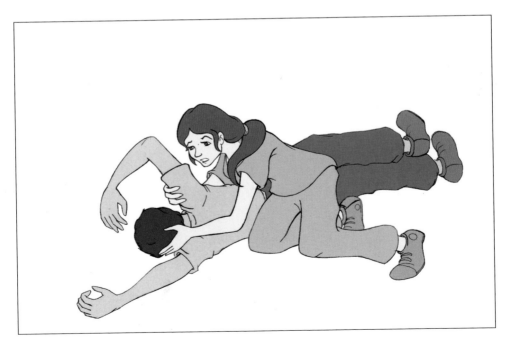

One-person log roll.

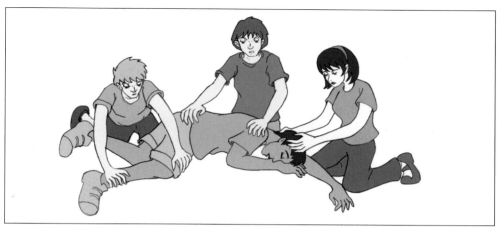

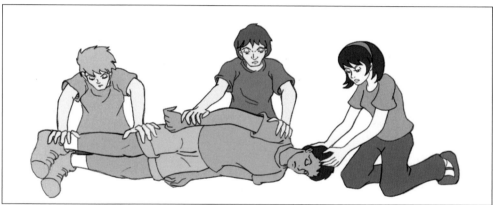

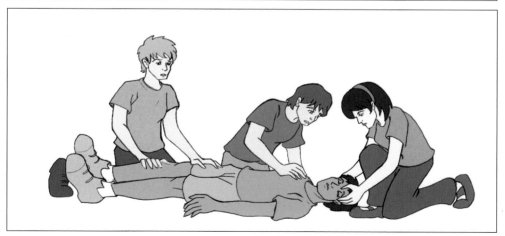

Two-person log roll.

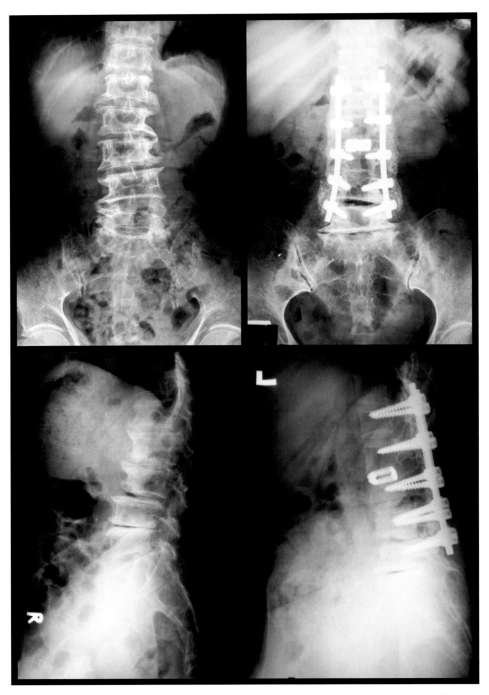

In the event of a spinal injury, evacuation is necessary so that a doctor can determine the source of the injury that may require surgical fixation.

- If there is any suspicion for cervical spinal injury, err on the side of caution with full immobilization and then necessary evacuation.

FOCUSED ASSESSMENT OF CERVICAL SPINE (FACS)

(Only perform if trained and comfortable with this procedure.)
- The patient is sober, alert, and cooperative.
- No strength deficits in hand grip, wiggling of fingers, and foot–push/pull.
- No sensation deficits in upper or lower limbs (sharp vs dull differentiation).
- No painful injury that may distract the patient from the presence of neck pain.
- No tenderness to pushing on the upper (neck) midline bony prominences.

CHECK YOUR FACS

If patient is alert, sober, has no point tenderness to midline neck vertebrae, has no sensation or motor deficits, and has no distracting painful injuries, *and* can rotate head 45 degrees to either shoulder, and touch chin to chest without pain in the middle of the neck (side of neck pain is okay, as this is likely from sore neck muscles), you can "clear" the upper spine without concern for a serious spinal injury or need for further neck immobilization.

Treatment
- Stabilize the spine by manually holding the head "in-line" with the rest of the body.
- Apply neck immobilization (e.g., molded SAM splint, backpack waist belt, etc.).
- Any log roll or movement done in small increments.
- If a litter is needed (*see* **Appendix B**), ensure to apply maximum padding around bony points and under knees and lower back with awareness of protection from the environment (e.g., cold, wet, sun, etc.) and removal of wet clothing.

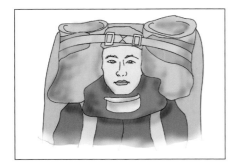
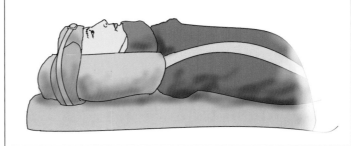

Improvised cervical spine immobilization.

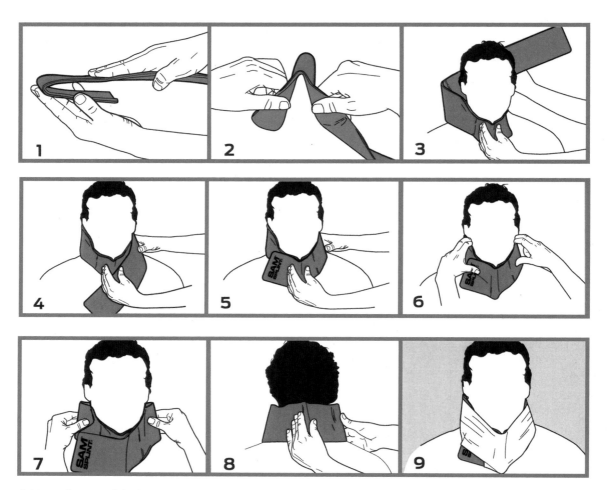

Evacuate: Any patient who has a possible spinal injury (cannot be cleared by FACS or cannot walk due to pain).

SAM splint molded cervical collar. *Images and splinting technique courtesy of SAM Medical.*

28
WOUND CARE

Most bleeding is obvious with a quick visual inspection. Blood from low pressure veins flowing out, and blood from arteries spurting out with the pumping heart, can be life-threatening. Controlling the bleeding may be the first step in the resuscitative care of an injured person. During the secondary assessment, be sure to check under a person's clothes with a hand sweep and look underneath them, to ensure there are no places of disguised blood loss.

Serious blood loss can occur internally from an injured organ or bleeding vessel that may not

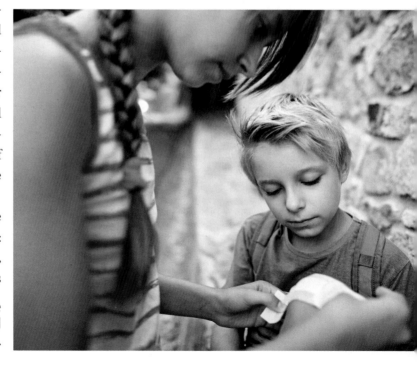

be visible or obvious. Always consider the MOI of the injury, and be aware of symptoms of progressive blood loss (e.g., dizziness exacerbated with sitting up or standing, rapid pulse, fatigue and weakness on exertion, and worsening pain and/or tenderness of the abdomen or other part of the body).

Wound management in the backcountry involves three steps: (1) control bleeding, (2) irrigation, and (3) wound closure. Always

Wound care is essential in the backcountry—even a small cut can get infected.

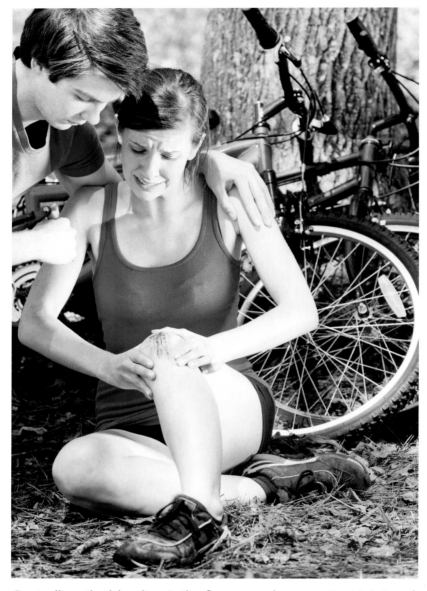

Controlling the bleeding is the first step when a patient is injured.

use gloves and universal precautions when dealing with body fluids to avoid transmission of blood borne diseases. Most wounds are simple and will stop with direct pressure and eleva-

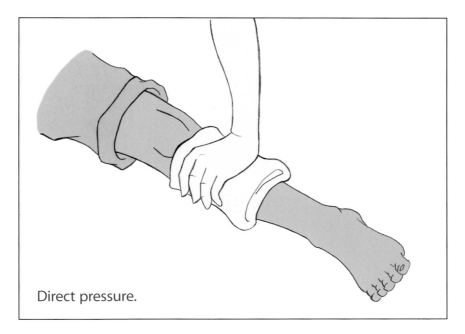

Direct pressure.

tion—very rarely are tourniquets indicated. Remember that any tourniquet may lead to eventual limb amputation, so use only as a last resort when life-threatening bleeding is occurring—when it's "Life or Limb." Any wound that occurs in the backcountry is at risk of getting infected. Copious irrigation and flushing out all visible foreign matter is the first step to minimizing poor outcomes. Any water that is safe to drink is safe to flush a wound with. Finally, closing a wound may optimize aesthetic outcome but increases the risk of infection. Wounds that are not closed should be packed with clean/sterile gauze and allowed to drain and heal on their own.

Treatment: Controlling Bleeding

- Direct pressure (on a small surface area, using a clean gauze bandage) for ten to fifteen minutes. Can use compressive wrap. The smaller the area of the compressive dressing directly on the wound, the greater the pressure exerted.
- If possible, elevate extremity above level of heart.
- Can apply a moist regular tea bag to wound to assist with bleeding control.
- If the patient has continued extremity bleeding despite the aforementioned methods, and there is concern that they may bleed to death, consider a tourniquet—"Life or Limb!"

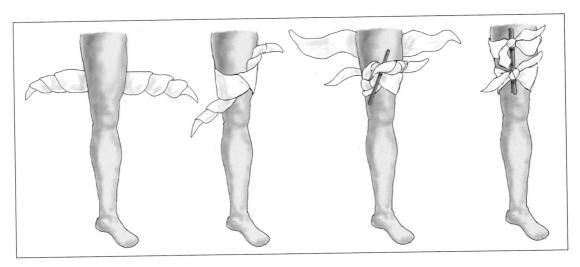

Tourniquet.

Tourniquet

1. Secure a band of cloth (at least two inches wide) two inches above extremity wound (between wound and the heart), as close to the lowest joint as possible. Do not place over the joint.

2. Tie half an overhand knot, put a small stick or rod on top of knot, and finish the half overhand knot over it The stick is the windlass that will tighten the tourniquet and provide mechanical advantage..

3. Tighten tourniquet by turning stick until bleeding stops. Secure the stick (tape or another cloth knot).

4. Loosen the tourniquet in twenty minutes to check for bleeding. If bleeding continues, reapply tourniquet and note time of application. If bleeding has stopped, leave tourniquet off.

Remember: Applying a tourniquet may result in limb amputation.

Treatment: Irrigation

• Irrigate the wound with forceful pressure with an irrigation syringe, drinking tube from a hydration bladder or sports bottle, or poke a hole (diameter

If water is safe to drink, then it is safe to irrigate a wound with.

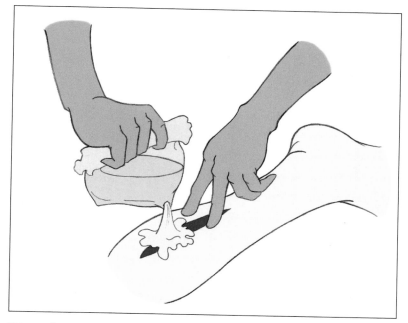

Wound irrigation.

of one safety pin) in the corner of a plastic bag, squeezing water out onto wound, using at least one liter of drinkable water.

- Pull wound edges apart for thorough cleaning.
- Abrasions should be scrubbed with soap and water.
- Any water safe to drink is safe to irrigate with.

Treatment: Wound Closure

- Wounds with edges that can be approximated may be closed: Use wound closure strips or paper tape to tape the wound shut. Apply tape perpendicular to wound, opposing the edges. Apply another piece of tape and/or benzoin adhesive perpendicular to anchor the strips.
- Cover with antibiotic ointment and gauze dressing.
- Change dressing every twenty-four hours.

Use gauze to cover the wound, and be sure to change the dressing every twenty-four hours.

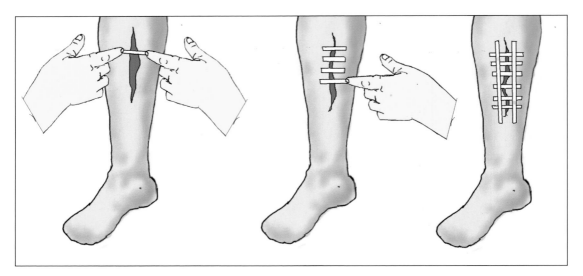

Wound closure.

- **Do Not Close:** puncture wounds, animal bites, or heavily contaminated wounds.
- Gaping or poorly opposed wounds may be left open to minimize infection. Apply antibiotic ointment (Bacitracin), cover with sterile/clean nonstick gauze, cover with gauze/wrap dressing.
- If wound is on joint of extremity, consider splinting wound.

⚠ **Red Flags:** Signs of infection, including pus, redness, streaking.

Treatment: Scalp Lacerations

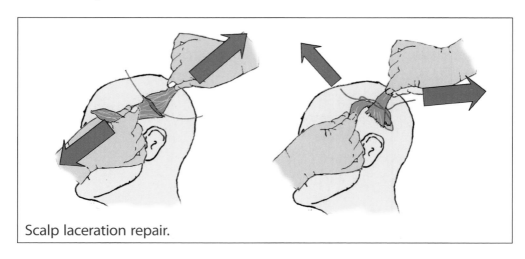

Scalp laceration repair.

- Take a strand of thread, fishing line, or thin string and lay it on top of (parallel to) the wound.
- Take strands of long hair on either side of the laceration and then cross them over, bringing the opposing wound edges together.
- Have another person tie a square knot with the thread as you hold the wound closed with hair.
- Repeat as many times as necessary down the length of the wound until the laceration is closed.

Treatment: Impaled Object

- Do not remove a large impaled object, as the object may be compressing and plugging shut injured tissues and its removal may lead to severe bleeding.
- Put a bulky dressing around the object to stabilize it.
- Secure the dressing well.
- Evacuate.

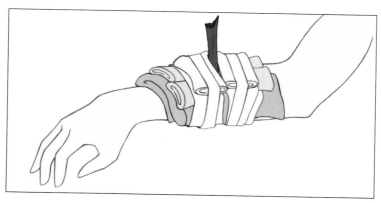

Impaled object.

Treatment: Embedded Fishhook

- Tie a string or shoelace around the bend of the hook.
- Push the shaft of the fishhook toward the barb/skin surface (this disengages the barb).
- Pull the string up and away at a 30-degree angle, yanking the hook from the skin with a snapping motion.

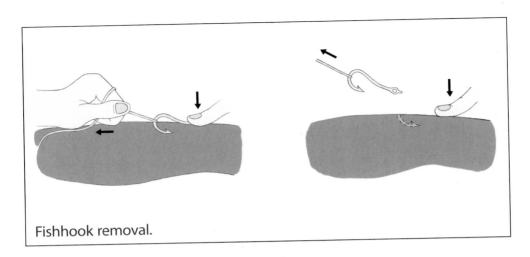

Fishhook removal.

Evacuate:

- Any amputation, tourniquet usage, or impaled object.
- Any wound that is heavily contaminated, is from a bite (human or animal), involves a joint space, or which may involve underlying tendons or ligaments (loss of range of motion of hand, foot, finger, or toe).
- Any wound infection.
- Any concern for hidden injury/internal bleeding.

APPENDIX A: MEDICATION INFORMATION

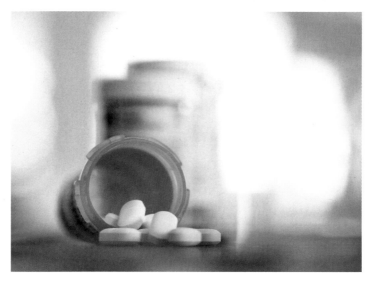

Only take prescription medication if you have been instructed by a physician or if someone's life is in danger without that medicine.

Do not provide prescription medicine unless you are a physician, have been instructed by a physician, or feel that someone's life is in danger if you do not give the medicine. Always ask about allergies prior to dispensing any medicine.

In addition to having medication administration protocols, you should obtain informed consent for medication administration, even nonprescription medication. Inform the recipient

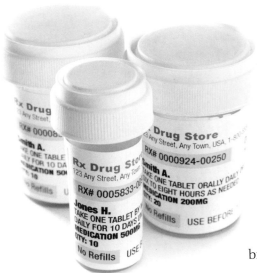

of the indications, contraindications, and possible side effects of the medication, and obtain consent to administer. Before administering any medication, read the protocols, confirm the dosage, read the label to confirm the medication, ask the patient about previous history with this medication and any known allergies, and ask the patient if he or she is currently on any other medications and, if so, review the protocols for contraindications.

All dosing is indicated for adults. Listed medicines as generic names as well as commonly encountered brand names.

Before administering medication, be sure to read the label for instructions and dosage.

ABBREVIATIONS

PO	Oral
IM	Intramuscular injection
OTC	Over-the-counter
Rx	Prescription

MEDICATION QUICK GUIDE

Pain Relief OTC

Acetaminophen	*(Tylenol)*
Ibuprofen	*(Advil, Motrin)*
Naproxen	*(Aleve)*

Anti-Allergy OTC

Hydrocortisone cream	
Diphenhydramine	*(Benadryl)*
Famotidine	*(Pepcid)*

Anti-Allergy Rx

Albuterol

Epinephrine   *(EpiPen)*

Antibiotic OTC

Polymyxin/bacitracin   *(Polysporin)*

Anti-Diarrheal OTC

Loperamide hydrochloride   *(Imodium)*

Bismuth subsalicylate   *(Pepto-Bismol)*

Anti-Nausea OTC

Famotidine   *(Pepcid)*

Bismuth subsalicylate   *(Pepto-Bismol)*

PAIN RELIEF OTC

Acetaminophen (Tylenol)

Classification: Non-narcotic pain relief, anti-fever.

Dose: See directions on label.

Indications: For relief of pain due to headache, cold, and flu discomfort, minor muscle and joint discomfort, and menstrual cramps. For reduction of fever. Especially useful for those allergic to aspirin or ibuprofen. Does not control inflammation.

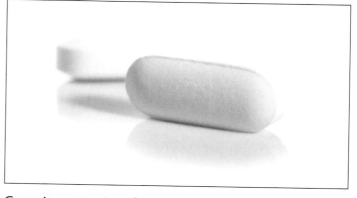

Generic acetaminophen.

Contraindications: Hypersensitivity, active alcoholism, liver disease, hepatitis. Acetaminophen is a common ingredient in over-the-counter pain, cold, and flu medicine. Be careful of accidental overdose in combination with other products.

Side Effects: Hypersensitivity rare.

Ibuprofen (Advil, Motrin)

Classification: Non-narcotic pain relief, anti-fever, non-steroidal anti-inflammatory.

Dose: See directions on label.

Indications: For symptomatic relief of pain associated with headache, colds, flu, frostbite, toothache, arthritis, burns, and menstrual cramps. May be used to reduce fever. For pain of inflammation and reduction of inflammation associated with muscle, joint, and over-use injuries. For prevention of acute mountain sickness and treatment of high altitude headache.

Contraindications: Active stomach or intestinal ulcer, gastrointestinal bleeding disorder, history of hypersensitivity to aspirin or other non-steroidal anti-inflammatory drugs.

Side Effects: Nausea, abdominal pain, dizziness, rash.

Naproxen (Aleve)

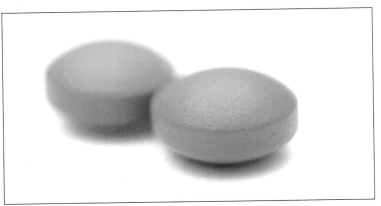

Generic ibuprofen.

Classification: Non-narcotic pain relief, anti-fever, non-steroidal anti-inflammatory.

Dose: See directions on label.

Indications: For relief of pain from headache, toothache, arthritis, muscle aches, tendinitis, and menstrual cramps. May be used to reduce fever and to treat pain of inflammation and reduction of inflammation associated with muscle, joint, and over-use injuries.

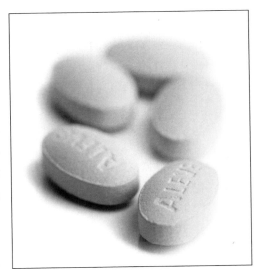

Aleve.

Contraindications: Active stomach or intestinal ulcer, gastrointestinal bleeding disorder, history of hypersensitivity to aspirin or other non-steroidal anti-inflammatory drugs.
Side Effects: Nausea, upset stomach, heartburn, headache, dizziness, drowsiness, bruising, and rash.

ANTI-ALLERGY OTC

Hydrocortisone cream
Classification: Glucocorticoid (steroid)
Dose: See directions on label.
Indications: For relief of pain and itching of jellyfish stings, poison ivy, oak, stinging nettles, sumac, insect bites, and other allergic skin reactions. May help dry up oozing rash of allergic skin reactions.
Contraindications: Infections.
Side Effects: Itching, redness, irritation
Diphenhydramine (Benadryl)
Classification: Antihistamine (H1-blocker)
Dose: For adults, 25–50mg/6 hours PO

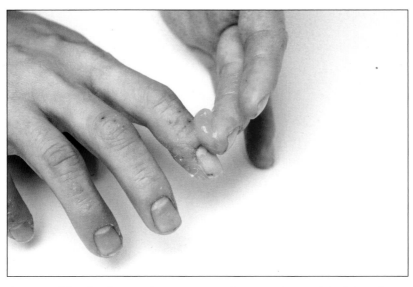

Creams like hydrocortisone can relieve pain and itching from allergic skin reactions.

Indications: For temporary relief of respiratory allergy symptoms and cold symptoms. Helps relieve the itching of allergic skin reactions. Useful in treatment of mild, moderate, and severe allergic and anaphylactic reactions. May be used as a mild sedative and for insomnia. May help alleviate seasickness.

Contraindications: Hypersensitivity, acute asthma attack, glaucoma, peptic ulcer.

Side Effects: Drowsiness, dizziness, weakness, dry mouth, thickening lung secretions, inability to urinate.

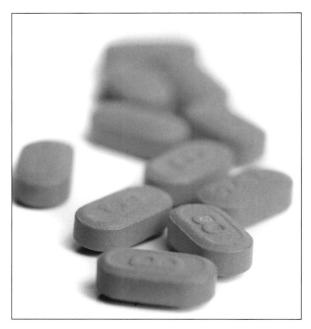

Benadryl.

Famotidine (Pepcid)

Classification: Antihistamine (H2-blocker)

Dose: See directions on label.

Indications: For heartburn, acid stomach, and ulcer disease. Useful in treatment of "sour stomach," and moderate and severe allergic and anaphylactic reactions.

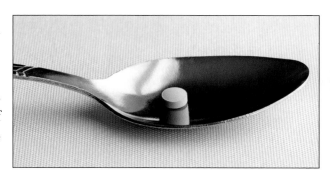

A famotidine pill.

Contraindications: Hypersensitivity to famotidine or other H2-blockers.
Side Effects: Constipation, diarrhea, dizziness, headache.

ANTI-ALLERGY RX

Albuterol
Classification: Bronchodilator
Dose: See directions on label.
Indications: Shortness of breath or breathing difficulty thought to be secondary to reactive airway disease (asthma) or anaphylaxis.
Contraindications: Fast heart rate secondary to underlying heart condition.
Side Effects: Palpitations, fast heart rate, tremor.

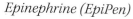

Albuterol can be administered through an inhaler.

Epinephrine (EpiPen)
Classification: Bronchodilator, antiallergenic, cardiac stimulant.
Dose: See directions on label.
Indications: For severe allergic reactions including anaphylaxis and severe asthma attack.
Contraindications: No true contraindications with anaphylaxis, hypertension, cardiac disease, glaucoma, shock.
Side Effects: Increased heart rate, nervousness, dizziness, lightheadedness, nausea, headache.

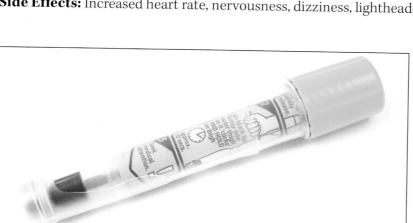

Follow directions to correctly and safely dispense epinephrine, often from an EpiPen.

ANTIBIOTIC OTC

Polymyxin B sulfate/bacitracin (Polysporin)

Classification: Antibiotic

Dose: See directions on label.

Indications: Contains ingredients for prevention of infection in minor wounds. Works as a lubricant, offers some relief from itching.

Contraindications: Hypersensitivity.

Side Effects: Hypersensitivity reactions: burning, itching, inflammation, contact dermatitis.

ANTI-DIARRHEAL OTC

Loperamide hydrochloride (Imodium)

Classification: Antidiarrheal

Dose: See directions on label.

Indications: For use in the control of diarrhea. Thought to limit peristalsis. Helpful in evacuating someone with severe diarrhea.

Contraindications: Hypersensitivity, bloody stool.

Side Effects: Dry mouth, dizziness, abdominal discomfort.

Bismuth subsalicylate (Pepto-Bismol)

Classification: Antidiarrheal

Dose: See directions on label.

Indications: For use in the control of diarrhea.

Contraindications: Hypersensitivity to aspirin.

Side Effects: Gray-black stool/tongue, nausea/vomiting, constipation, ringing in ears.

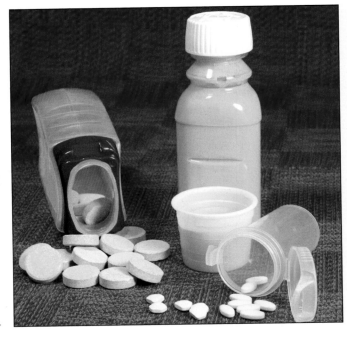

Pepto-Bismol comes in both liquid and tablet form.

ANTI-NAUSEA OTC

Bismuth subsalicylate (Pepto-Bismol) chewable tablets

Classification: Anti-diarrheal.

Dose: See directions on label.

Indications: For use in the control of nausea.

Contraindications: Hypersensitivity to aspirin.

Side Effects: Gray-black stool/tongue, nausea/vomiting, constipation, ringing in ears.

Famotidine (Pepcid)

Classification: Antihistamine (H2-blocker).

Dose: See directions on label.

Indications: For heartburn, "sour stomach," and ulcer disease. Can be used in conjunction with Phenergan for nausea. Useful in treatment of moderate allergic and anaphylactic reactions.

Contraindications: Hypersensitivity to famotidine or other H2-blockers.

Side Effects: Constipation, diarrhea, dizziness, headache.

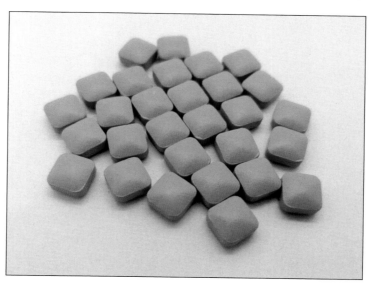

Another kind of famotidine pill.

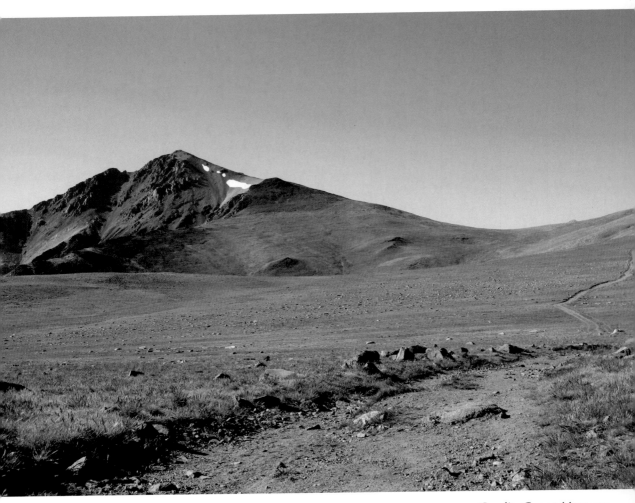

Credit: Grant Lipman

APPENDIX B: EVACUATION INFORMATION

One of the most difficult decisions in wilderness medicine is whether to evacuate a victim. Not only is an evacuation prematurely ending an adventure, but as there is often substantial money, time, and training that went into the trip planning, there are multiple variables at risk of being lost. But safety needs to be the top priority. Be aware of the "red flags" for the disease process in play, and early preparation and planning will be an advantage before issues progress. It is preferable to assist someone during the day than to extricate them with a stretcher at night! A potential evacuation is an undertaking with multiple hazards that need to be taken into account prior to embarking: changing environmental conditions, maneuvering an injured person over inclement terrain, worsening of the victim's condition, and support for and needs of the rescuers.

EVACUATION TIPS

- Remember to have shelter. Evacuations take longer than expected, so prepare for an overnight bivouac or unexpected weather. As a French mountain guide once told me in the Karakorum, "You could die up there. Bring a tent."
- If you send a messenger to get help, write down the salient medical and logistical information so the rescuers can both locate and bring appropriate resources.
- It is next to impossible to carry any but the lightest victim over any substantial distances. For example, it takes six to eight trained rescuers to extricate an adult. While the

concept of a litter system or rope carry is attractive, exhausting the rescuers from futile attempts will not benefit anyone.

- If using an improvised stretcher, make it as comfortable as possible—you cannot use enough padding.
- Remember empathy. There are limited resources available in the wilderness first-aid kit to treat the hurt and fear of the victim. Often the most useful tools are reassurance, commiseration, and empathy. The rescuer suddenly has the responsibility of a dependent who may be incapacitated, and it is reasonable to assign an individual in the rescue party to look out for the victim's needs (e.g. hunger, thirst, toilet, and comfort, etc.).

DAISY CHAIN LITTER SYSTEM

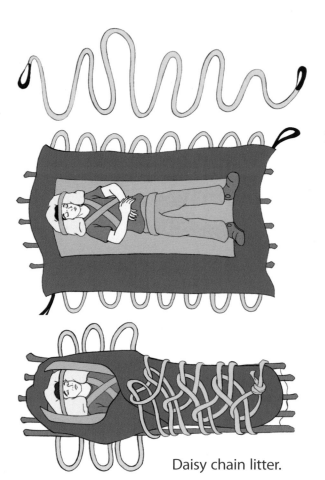

Daisy chain litter.

Materials needed:
- Rope, at least eighty feet (twenty-five meters) long.
- Tarp or tent fly.
- Sleeping bag or sleeping pad.

Instructions:
1. Lay out the daisy chain; loops are arms' width (six feet), with fifteen to twenty loops.

2. Lay tarp and/or padding on the rope and package the patient.

3. Tie a loop knot with a bight (figure 8) at the foot end of the rope. Wrap the patient, cinching and looping each successive length towards the head, then tie off the rope.

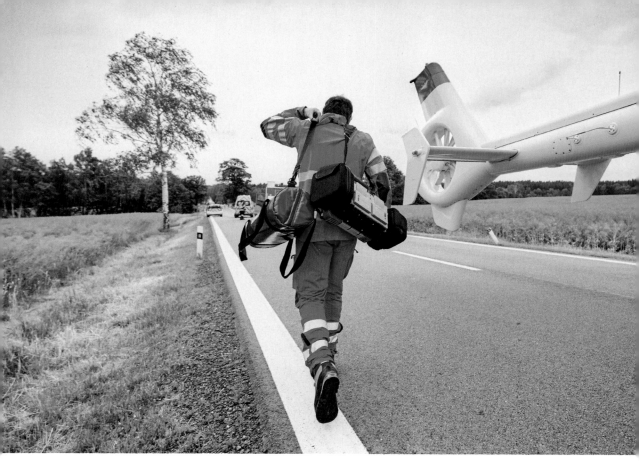

If a patient has a better chance of recovery with an air evacuation, a helicopter evacuation can be considered.

HELICOPTER RESCUE AND SAFETY

Conditions for Helicopter Evacuation

- The victim's chances of recovery are better with air than they are with ground evacuation.
- A ground evacuation would be arduous or unduly dangerous to either victim or the rescuers.
- The helicopter pilot and crew would be functioning within their safety protocols.

Information for Helicopter Team

- Number of patients.
- Patients' weight and medical status.
- Wind direction at landing zone.

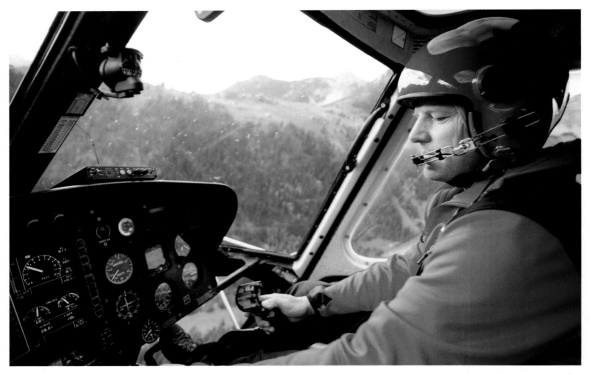

The helicopter pilot must operate within their safety protocols during an evacuation.

- Weather conditions at landing zone.
- UTM or latitude/longitude coordinates and altitude.
- Geographical description of landing zone.

Do-Not-Fly Conditions

- Winds over 40 mph (70 Km/hr).
- Night flight into mountainous areas.
- Low visibility.
- Poor or unknown landing conditions.
- Slopes of more than 10 degrees.

Safety Rules

- Never approach a helicopter until signaled to do so by the pilot or crew.
- Keep in line-of-sight view of the pilot and crew.
- Clear away debris prior to helicopter approach, then stay clear of the landing zone.

- Stand outside landing zone with back to the wind, facing the approach.
- Approach from downhill.
- *Do not* approach from uphill.
- Avoid the tail rotor.

Landing Zone Set-Up

- Day: 100 feet x 100 feet (thirty big paces).
- Night: 150 feet x 150 feet (fifty big paces).
- Mark location/corners of landing zone with brightly colored objects/clothes that can show wind direction.

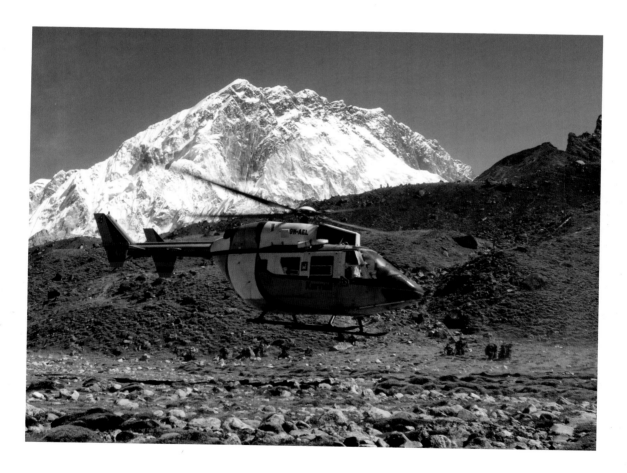

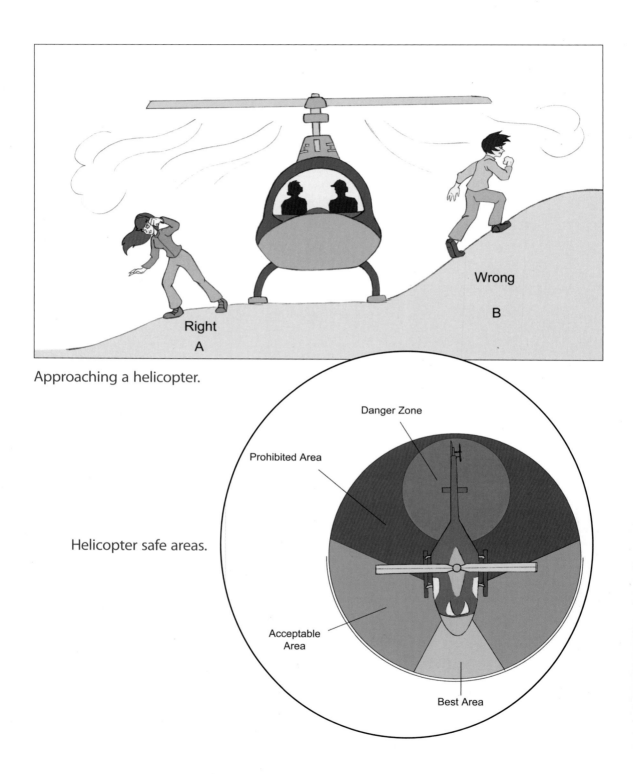

Approaching a helicopter.

Helicopter safe areas.

Danger Zone

Prohibited Area

Acceptable Area

Best Area

Right

A

Wrong

B

APPENDIX C: FIRST AID KIT

BASIC FIRST-AID KIT

- √ SAM splint
- √ Scissors
- √ Safety pins
- √ Duct tape
- √ Wound closure strips (¼" x 4")
- √ Benzoin (liquid adhesive) prep pads
- √ Alcohol prep pads
- √ Elastikon (3")
- √ Paper tape
- √ Spenco 2nd Skin (1" pads)
- √ Latex or nitrile gloves
- √ CPR microshield mask
- √ Cotton swabs
- √ 4" x 4" gauze dressing
- √ Compression bandage wrap
- √ Sunblock

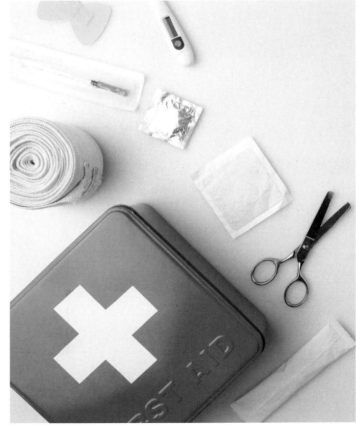

Bring a first-aid kid when you travel into the wilderness.

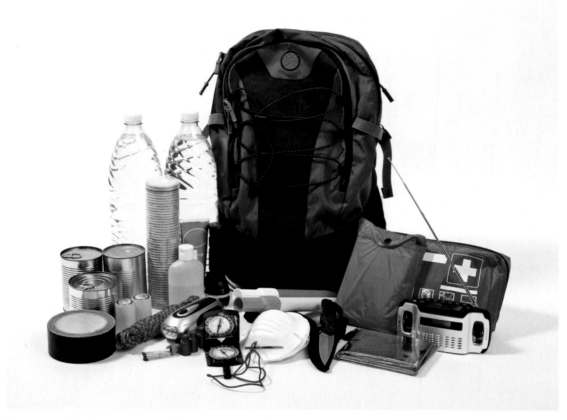

Prepare all of your survival essentials before going on a wilderness outing.

SURVIVAL ESSENTIALS

√ Emergency space blanket
√ Whistle
√ Water bottle and water purification system
√ Food
√ Headlamp and batteries
√ Map/compass/GPS
√ Fire starter system
√ Signal mirror
√ Appropriate clothes/rain shell
√ Parachute cord (4 mm or ³⁄₁₆")—50 feet

NOTES

NOTES

NOTES

NOTES

NOTES

NOTES

NOTES

NOTES